SAILING **ON BROKEN PIECES**

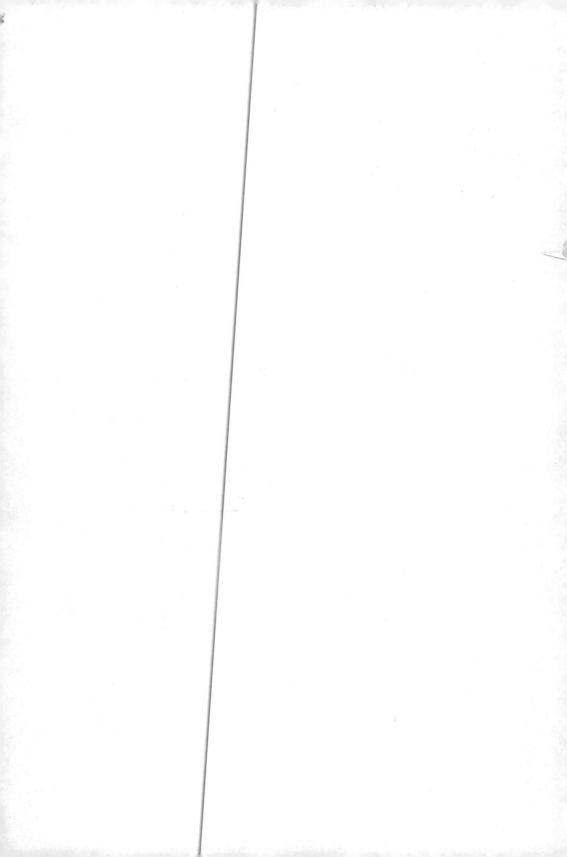

SAILING
ON BROKEN PIECES

Essential Survival Skills for Recovery from Mental Illness

GARY RHULE

NEW YORK

SAILING **ON BROKEN PIECES**
Essential Survival Skills for Recovery from Mental Illness

Published in New York, New York, by Morgan James Publishing. Morgan James and The Entrepreneurial Publisher are trademarks of Morgan James, LLC.
www.MorganJamesPublishing.com

The Morgan James Speakers Group can bring authors to your live event. For more information or to book an event visit The Morgan James Speakers Group at www.TheMorganJamesSpeakersGroup.com.

The poem, *Different*, is used with permission of the poet, Donna Wilkinson Maxwell.

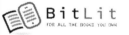

BitLit
FOR ALL THE BOOKS YOU OWN

FREE eBook edition for your existing eReader with purchase

PRINT NAME ABOVE

For more information, instructions, restrictions, and to register your copy, go to **www.bitlit.ca/readers/register** or use your QR Reader to scan the barcode:

ISBN 978-1-61448-942-9 paperback
ISBN 978-1-61448-943-6 eBook
ISBN 978-1-61448-945-0 hardcover
Library of Congress Control Number:
2013948910

Cover Design by:
Rachel Lopez
www.r2cdesign.com

Interior Design by:
Bonnie Bushman
bonnie@caboodlegraphics.com

In an effort to support local communities, raise awareness and funds, Morgan James Publishing donates a percentage of all book sales for the life of each book to Habitat for Humanity Peninsula and Greater Williamsburg.

Get involved today, visit
www.MorganJamesBuilds.com

Habitat
for Humanity®
Peninsula and
Greater Williamsburg
Building Partner

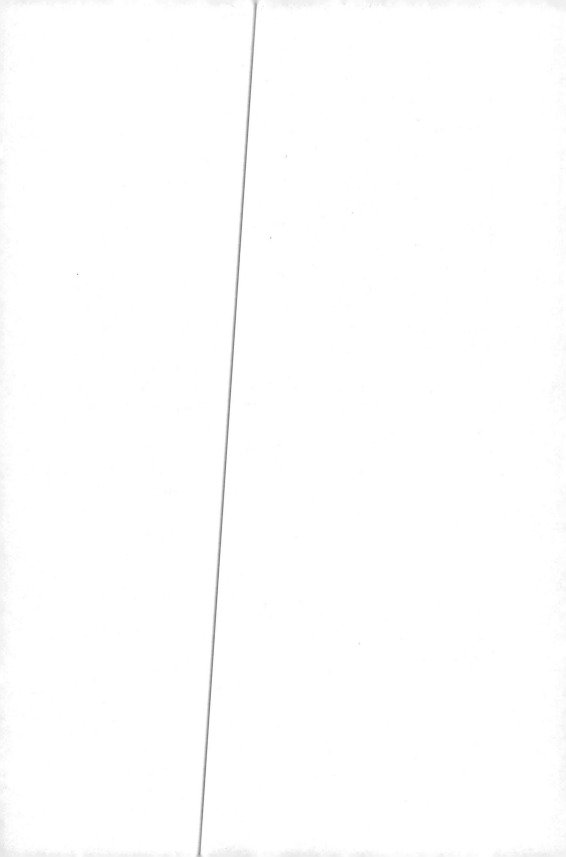

For my brother

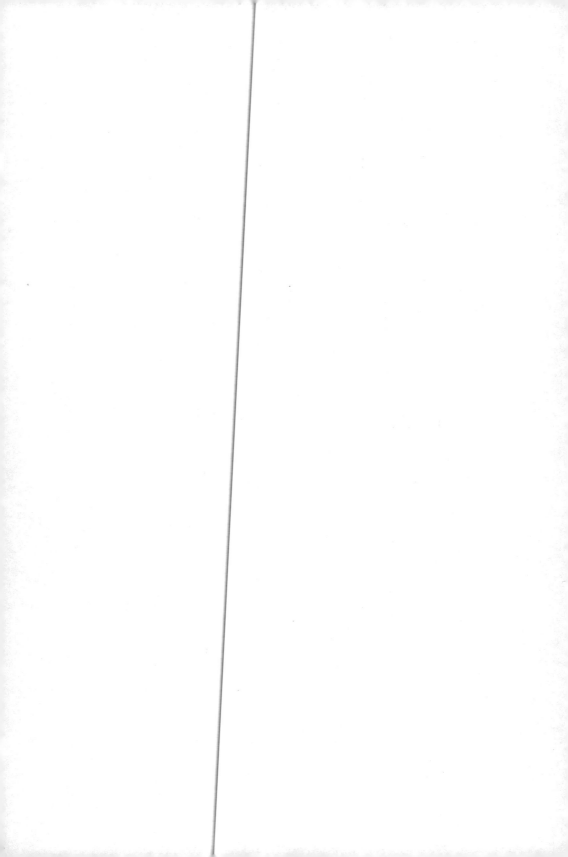

CONTENTS

ACKNOWLEDGMENTS

I am deeply thankful to my mother, father, and sisters for their unwavering support. Without their encouragement, this book would not have been possible.

In memory of my grandparents who lifted me up, and allowed me to stand on their shoulders, so that I could see farther than I could while alone.

I am grateful to the friends who loudly cheered me on while writing, who told me it was possible, and kept me focused so that it could be completed. They include Deborah M. Grogan, Ian Hinds, Steven A. Smith, Donna Wilkinson Maxwell, Jeffrey A. Stewart, Maxcine C. Howell, Troy Stewart, Annette Sanderson, Sharon Walker, Roya Rezai, and Wayne Fuller.

A special thanks to Pat Miller for timely inspiration and words of wisdom for the book's title. To Lenny Thompson who showed me the power of positive thought. I must also give special thanks to Barbara Strong Wiggins and Francesca Borges Gordon for their encouragement to keep on writing when I was facing a roadblock. They helped me to appreciate the power of kindness in every spoken word and to return it to others.

For the individuals, clinicians, and health care providers, for the random acts of kindness that they bestowed on my brother, we are deeply thankful.

I also wish to thank the many family caregivers of persons with mental illness, who work in silence and help their loved ones to mental health recovery, and who in their everyday lives work to remove the stigma of mental illness.

And the rest, some on boards,
and some on broken pieces of the ship.
And so it came to pass,
that they escaped all safe to land.
Acts 27:44.

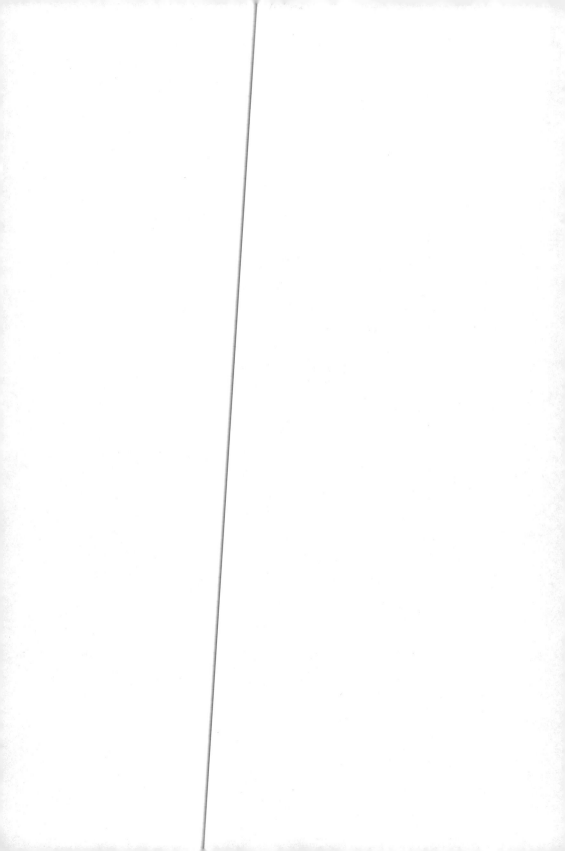

PROLOGUE:

THE WIND SAID NO

I only wanted to be free.

I desperately wanted to be released from this life that was not my own.

I knew that was not possible so I stifled the primal scream that was bubbling up from my inner core. That scream had been simmering and building up pressure for quite some time now. I wanted to go to the tiptop of a mountain, any mountain, any high building, or even to the nearest high point that I could see. I needed to yell and yell, scream and scream, do something, just anything, to release the tension and pressure. Every fiber of my body needed that release. I needed to let it all out so that I could simply breathe and simply be free.

Despite the adrenaline that flooded my body I consciously tried to slow down my heartbeat. I was trying to suppress something that was completely subconscious and that was controlled by my mind. Nevertheless, I had to stop this feeling because if there were no release or no suppression of the tension, I did not know what would happen. But, I had to do something; otherwise soon I would be trembling and sweating. I felt like I would succumb to the pressure and explode. If I got to that point, would I too lose control of my own mind and my body?

I clenched my fists and took deep gulps of fresh air into my lungs and breathed. I felt like the first time that I had gone swimming and put my face in the water. I had held my breath too long because I was scared to start to breathe while under the water. However, I had held my breath for too long. When I was forced to stand up to catch my breath, the loud gasp for air was cacophonous and it expelled from my mouth with such force that all the other swimmers in and out of the pool looked around to see if I were drowning. I was drowning. But when I exhaled and sucked deeply on that vital need for oxygen, my heart's beat was calmed, and that helped to nourish my brain so that my entire body would calm down just a little bit for me to stop trembling. I became a little calmer.

In spite of that, I felt that I was still driving frantically down Main Street. I was hyped, vigilant, and ready. I was in ready-set-go mode, and ready to confront whatever or whomever I had to so that I could bring this thing to conclusion.

I glanced from side to side at the sidewalks and into the bus stop shelters. My vision was sharp, but I could barely make out the people's faces. They were walking much too fast trying to get somewhere quickly. Anywhere. They crouched into their jackets to escape the cold and the wind. The outside temperature was dropping fast. It foretold a sinister fall season and an even colder than usual winter. I could not see into the future, but every event took on some uncanny meaning.

None of these people even looked like Sam, my brother. If he was anywhere close to this place, I should be able to make him out. He was tall, thin, and limped to the right when he walked. It should not be that difficult to make him out in any crowd. Maybe I was driving by too quickly to see him. Despite being on edge and super-alert, it was not working to my advantage.

"Slow the car down. Slow the car down. Drive slower. That way you can get a better look at what's around you. You will be able to see better," I told myself.

"Where is he, anyway?"

Only several minutes before my cell phone would not stop ringing. At first, I wanted to ignore it, but when I looked at the caller ID, I saw that it was Charlie. Charlie had been persistent. It must have been important, and it was. Charlie had been trying to call me to say that Sam had not returned yet.

"Dr. Gary, Sam has not come back in," Charlie said into the phone.

"What do you mean?" I asked.

"Well, it is 7:45 in the evening, and you know, curfew is 9 p.m. He has not come back in," Charlie said calmly.

"Huh? What? What's that? Okay. Well, what time did he leave there today?" I asked trying not to sound ticked off.

"Ah. Ah. He left about nine this morning to go to his appointment at the center," Charlie said.

"Well, it is 7:45 in the evening now and obviously, Sam would not be there. The center has to be closed by now as they do not have appointments after 5 p.m. No one would be there now. Did the other patients come back already?"

"Yeah, yeah. They all came back around one o'clock," Charlie said again very calmly.

"So, did you ask Isaac if he saw him?" I thought had he called and asked everyone before he had called me? Why did it take more than six hours after Sam should have come back for him to call me anyway?

"Yeah, you mean his buddy Izzie?" Charlie asked. Isaac was called Izzie by his friends, and I had asked to be sure because I was thinking that Charlie had not done any of that.

"Of course, who else?" I thought. "How many other Izzie's do you know that is Sam's buddy?" I decided not to say any of that out loud because serving ice in response to calmness would not be too cool.

"Yes, yes. Did you ask Izzie if he saw him?" I repeated, and tried not to make my voice sound chipped and sharp like the edges of ice sometimes become.

"Yes. I asked him and Izzie said he had not seen Sam at all today."

"Well, didn't Marlon take him this morning to the center?" I asked now audibly annoyed.

"No. Remember? You know they said he was okay to take the bus," Charlie replied. "Don't you remember?"

"Remember? Remember? Who can remember all that stuff?" I wondered.

"They are at it again," I muttered.

"And in fact, Charlie, I don't remember any of that. I have a good memory and I don't recall any of that," I said quietly to myself. I remember faces well but I may not remember your name. Faces stuck in my memory even if I had trouble recalling the time and place where we had met. Otherwise though, my memory was pretty good and I don't remember them telling me that Sam was well enough now to be independent and to take a bus home alone.

"Well, I guess I have to go find him right?" I asked.

"Right? Right?" I repeated because obviously Charlie had not heard me the first time around.

Charlie did not even respond. He chose not to respond.

"I will call you when I find him and call you right back. Thanks," I said.

"Well, thanks for nothing," I said to myself, staring at the cellphone in my hand. I was breathing too shallowly now, and it felt like I was holding my breath again, and I could hardly breathe.

That was surely great help. Charlie must have hung up the phone. I did not stop to listen to hear if he had said goodbye or goodnight or good riddance or good whatever. He did not say, "Okay, I will wait for your call." The line simply had gone dead, and I continued to stare at the cell phone in my hand.

My chest was starting to hurt as I must have breathed too deeply that time. I was hurting my ribs by holding my breath too long and then breathing too deeply on the next breath.

"Okay, okay. I got this, I got this," I said over and over to calm myself down. It's not like it is the end of creation and the world was coming to an end. The earth had lived through the ice age and survived. But I was really tired of feeling like it was trial and error over and over. But any reaction now would still get me going in the right direction, right?

I breathed, this time a little more deeply. I had then grabbed my car keys, gotten in my car, and driven out to Main Street to begin the search.

There was nothing on Main Street, nothing. No sign of Sam. I did not even know what he had been wearing today. I knew I had to be calm. But the more I drove, the more I felt the pressure. The tension was there and I knew I needed more adrenaline to keep on going. I must find him and find him now, therefore, I steadied my thoughts, slowed the racing of my mind, and forced myself to think more clearly.

"Okay, he must not have come down Main Street at all as I had not seen him walking. What bus would he have taken?" I wondered.

He would have had to go downtown first as that was the bus route he was on. And then he would need to transfer buses when he got downtown. He would then need to come back up Albany Avenue in the same direction from which he had just left. In my state of mind, I did not understand the logic of the bus route, and to tell the truth, I didn't really care at this point.

They said he was safe to take the bus to the center. I wondered if when all this blew over, if the bus routes would make any sense what-so-ever to me or to anyone else. Why you could not simply have a path that took you across the bottom of what would have been a triangle to get to your destination. It would have been straight, simple, and logical. But, they made nothing simple and they simply could not make anything easy. Sometimes when you are mired in the midst of a situation, you cannot make sense of the logic and pattern that was clearly before you. You paid so much attention to the muck that you were in that you forgot to look up, and look out, and see that there was a plan and a design for what was happening. You only had to take the time and the energy to look up, and make the connections, and see the intricacies in the design and plan.

"Oh, God, Sam is nowhere in sight," I moaned.

"Where is he?"

I drove to the mental health center. The center was a single story concrete block building, weather-beaten, and washed in a drab beige color. The signage identifying the building had what was meant to be a complementary dark brown background. The signage letters were spelled out in light blue, and there was a small light at the base of the sign shining on it so that you could read the lettering in the dark. The beige building had flood lights everywhere, and the lighting was fairly good all around the building. There were two entrances at the front of the building, one on the left and the other on the right.

The building was closed and that was obvious as all the lights inside were off. No one was around and not a single living soul was in sight. Hey, but why not double check? Better yet, I wanted to triple check, just in case. I stopped the car in the middle of the street and I walked to the bus shelter that was located near the front of the building. I peered inside to see who and what was in there but, I only found an empty bench inside. Sam was not in there sleeping and nothing and no one else was in there. My heart started to race but my legs were steady. My chest burned. I decided to walk up the wheelchair accessible ramp to get to the front entrance door on the left. I avoided the five steps to conserve as much energy as I could, as I did not know if I would be up all night looking for Sam, or dealing with whatever condition I found him in.

"Conserve your energy as you will need it."

He wasn't here.

"Stop, breathe, and think. Stop and think for a minute."

"Maybe you missed him when you were driving on Main Street? Were you even looking well enough?" I asked myself.

"What is he wearing today?" I said to the wind.

"If you knew what he wore today, that would help," the wind said.

It was now getting into the colder fall season and I still had not brought the heavier fall jacket to the assisted living center. I was tempted to toss out my check-list of to-do items. It was getting too long. I would complete five tasks and it was still growing. The jacket was somewhere lost on the list.

"Yeah, right, supposedly assisted living," I snorted in disgust.

"This was assisted living. Where was the assistance?" I complained.

"Well, I did not feel too assisted today. Is this what assistance looks like?"

If they had assisted, my check-list should have been much shorter. I decided to toss the check-list into the garbage the first chance I got. This list did not help me to focus on my top three priorities. It only added more stress to my life. My first tip was to toss the completely useless check-list out. Everything cannot be a priority, there is no such thing. I needed to remember to only do three things daily, tops. Nothing else should come on the short-list unless something was completed and came off. Nothing.

My mind was revved trying to figure out what Sam would have been wearing today. In the confusion of everything, I had not focused and just stuck to the basics. Why had I not seen him on any of the streets that I had just driven from? Had he walked another way and I had just missed him? Maybe he had already returned to the assisted living center, and I was just now only wasting good gas, and very precious time, and it would all be in vain.

"Oh. Oh. There is an ambulance stopped over there."

"Gary, stop and see what's up with them. If it is none of your business you can just press on."

My knuckles and fingers felt like they were frostbitten as I tightened my grip on the car's steering wheel. My chest cried out.

"No, no, no!" I screamed and struck the steering wheel with clenched fists.

"I have come too far now to fail," I said to the wind. "Please, I can't fail now!"

"No, no, no!" I repeated.

"Is this really a lost cause? Do I just run away and go live my own life? Do I give up now after putting in so much time and so much effort?" I asked.

"No, no, no," the wind answered.

"Okay," I said to myself enough to calm down, slowing my racing heartbeat and bringing back the blood to my hands. I steadied my mind and focused on the task at hand.

You heard the wind.

The wind said "No."

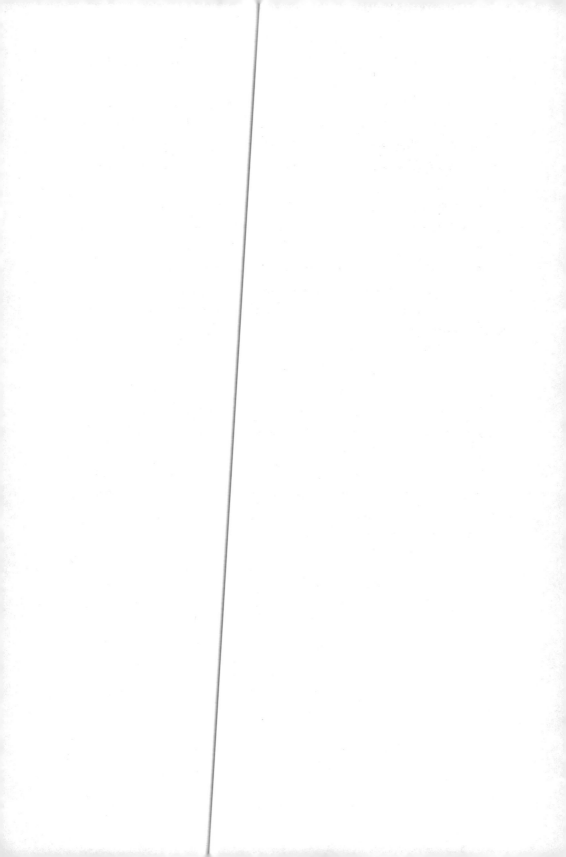

PART I

REFLECTIONS
IN THE WATER

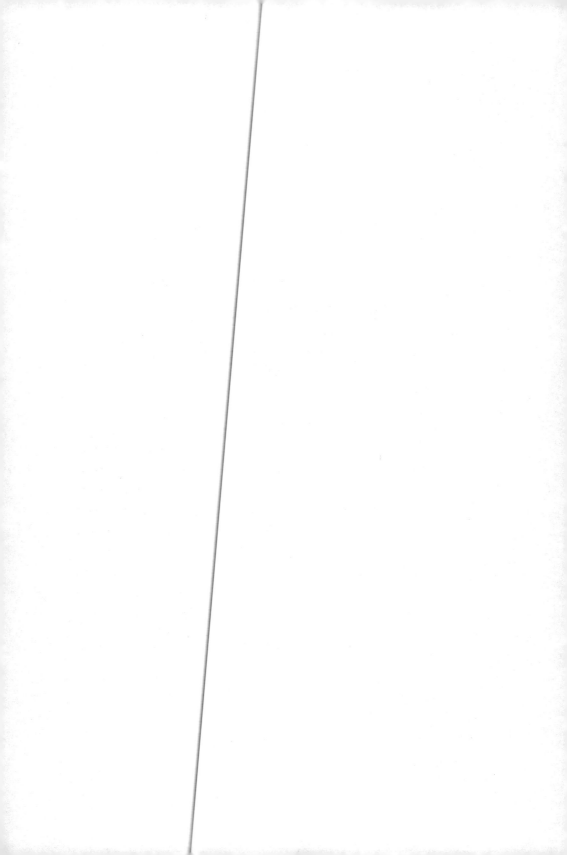

CHAPTER 1

THE HARDY BOYS

"Hey. Dr. Gary. Hey you," Paloma said to get my attention.

"Dr. Gary, you must come to Room 10 now," Paloma ordered. She held her shoulders and body straight up just as you would expect any commanding officer to stand. Paloma Bean was the charge nurse working the 3 p.m. to 11 p.m. shift tonight. She ran a tight ship, and it was a welcomed relief when she worked. She had many years of work experience in the emergency room. She looked younger than what I imagined was her actual age. But, I suspected that she dyed her hair to hide the gray streaks that tumbled out from what must have once been intensely blond locks. Her facial features were sharp. She had no crow feet at the eye lines, probably from never smiling at all. She probably had succumbed to a surgeon's knife to sculpt a youthful look.

Paloma was pulling with such force on my newly laundered white labcoat that she dragged me off the stool that I was sitting on at my workstation. At that point I had no choice but to move and to come with her. Paloma's face was emotionless. She simply needed me to be in another place right now and she intended to get me there even if it were against my will.

I lurched forward, but steadied myself before I would have slipped and have fallen. Paloma was yanking on my lab-coat so that I would come at once and deal with whatever and whoever was in Room 10. She didn't give me a chance to click out of the current screen in which I was working on the computer. My stethoscope was already slung around my neck; therefore, I was at least somewhat prepared for anything in the room. This must have been a real emergency for her to topple me off my chair like that.

The patient in Room 10 was Mr. Iguzi, and he was lying flat on the stretcher. He was obviously in pain, but he was very calm, and he did not move. I wondered if he was trying to center himself and work from an internal pain control center that he could manipulate and call on when it was needed. I wished I could draw on some internal energy source at all times to heal myself and not feel any pain. I wanted to be able to meditate even in the midst of chaos and remain calm and in control of my emotions and feelings.

Paloma said, "Hey, he fell, look at his right ankle. The paramedics already gave him something for pain in the ambulance."

"They placed an intravenous line already while coming to the emergency room," she continued.

"But, look at that, he needs more medication. He has no allergies, and his blood pressure is holding with the pain medications. I will go get some more of the same for him," she said as she turned to leave the room.

She ran down to the PYXIS machine to get the medication. She has been working the emergency room for twenty years yet, she was always pumped up in this hectic, fast-paced environment. She was one of those adrenaline junkies who loved being in the thick of everything and having her finger on the pulse of it all.

Paloma punched in her access codes and the PYXIS machine's door clicked open. She grabbed a vial of the drug and quickly ran back to the room.

"Look at that ankle," she said again.

"He fell off a ladder trying to reach up to clear the leaves from his gutters on the roof at his house."

I had already lifted the sterile cover that she had neatly placed over the right ankle so that I could look at it.

"Oh, oh," I said out more loudly than I had intended. I suppressed a wave of nausea that threatened to bubble up from my belly.

Mr. Iguzi's right ankle and foot looked like a mangled dinner fork. The foot was practically dangling off its hinges. The tibia, the larger bone in the lower leg, was sticking right out of the muscles and skin. All the bones and tissues of the ankle and foot were displayed for the entire world to see. Frank Netter, the medical illustrator, could have drawn the ankle's anatomy from this wide open view.

Surprisingly, there was little blood despite the magnitude of the injury. The lower part of the leg was completely open, broken, and obviously dislocated. I shook by body in disbelief as I imagined seeing him falling, and hearing the snap and loud crack as he fell off the ladder.

I suppressed the wave of nausea—one that your body experiences when slammed by intense pain. Most of us cannot tolerate intense pain, one that is so unbearable it pushes you to the edge. It brings with it a sudden wave of nausea that is followed by uncontrolled vomiting, sweating, and trembling. But, Mr. Iguzi was extremely calm. The body's own natural pain killer, the endorphins, must have kicked in and taken over to get him to a place of calm and quiet euphoria.

I was not that stoic. I would have screamed out loudly to relieve the pain, to expel it from my body. I don't think that I would have been that calm when faced with my own unbearable pain. But, I think that we are stronger than we believe. We find the courage and strength inside us to deal with the unbearable, even when we doubt that it is there in the first place. But, remember, it is in there.

"Remember?" That's what Charlie said to me yesterday. "Remember?"

Ankles

…Crack, crack, crack…

"One dark…"

…Crack, crack, crack…crack…

Gasterre brought the cane down onto his back with all her might and Sam's body racked and trembled with pain. Gasterre deliberately struck with all her strength so that the pain would transmit to every part of Sam's body. That was her intent. The power of the strike splintered on impact and transmitted itself to every morsel, every nook and cranny, in the skinny boy's body. The intensity of the pain slammed into Sam's back and rippled upward into his head and down into his toes. It did not lose its intensity as it meandered from the epicenter in his back to the other parts of his body. Every part of his body quivered and trembled as it struggled to find a new resting rhythm and an equilibrium that had existed immediately before the unexpected onslaught of the trauma brought on by the caning.

...Crack, crack, crack...

Sam refused to cry. Why cry today? He made up his mind not to cry today. He tensed all the muscles in his body, closed his eyes, and imagined that he was not in this place, not in this classroom. No, there was no way that he was going to cry today. He had done it before. He had willed away the urge to cry. If he dared, he would have moved his hands to cover his ears. If he could not hear Gasterre, and if he could not see her by keeping his eyes tightly shut, she would disappear from this place and be gone. If that did not work, he would just hold the tears in. He could live with the pain and bear it. In the Roadrunner, the runner fell off cliffs, was blown to smithereens, and simply got up and went on to the next disaster. Sam's thoughts raced uncontrollably and ransacked his mind. He could not focus on any one thought. The pain was intense, and he wanted to disappear into the bench that he sat on. If he could not disappear into it, then he wanted Gasterre just to be gone already. If he could sit here and take the pain then the world would know that he was strong. He wanted to be strong and not weak. He secretly vowed to himself never to cry and he would try not to.

"One dark night...it's you, it's you, you know, man..."

"One dark night, when...when...it's you, it's you, you know, man..."

Crack, crack, crack...

"Read!" Gasterre commanded.

Sam hated the classroom. Nothing seemed to make sense to him here. The words on the page appeared jumbled. If Gasterre would only stop the yelling, he could concentrate on one thing at a time, and figure out what to do. There were just too many steps to follow and too many things to remember all at once. He did much better in the mathematics class as the counting and adding up numbers was easier than reading.

"Now, read!"

"You are as dumb as a rock!" Gasterre yelled. "Now, read!"

"One dark night, when it was…it's you, it's you, you know, man…."

Crack…crack…

The cane continued to savagely rain down licks across Sam's back. He could not do both, holding the tears in and reading out loud. Gasterre did not care for she wanted Sam for once to be able to read the lesson for the day, any lesson. Just at least this once, to read and read correctly all that was on the page. Sam knew deep down that he was not going to be strong today.

Crack…crack…

Not today…today was supposed to be the day to be strong, but it was not going to happen today.

Crack…crack…crack…

Sam screamed out in pain and allowed the tears to freely flow down his face. He tasted the salt and licked the tears as they splattered on his face. He licked his lips. His nose started to run and the nasal contents flung itself out of its confinement and onto the floor. In less than thirty seconds his shirt was soaked, and the floor around him had gobs of white creamy congealing nasal discharge on the classroom's floor. Sam thought that Gasterre was trying to kill him. Looking at the dampness on his shirt and the mess on the floor, he thought that she almost succeeded. Sam stood there with his head hanging down. Gasterre was still waiting for him to read out loud. Sam relished the salt and tears and the draining nasal contents and closed his eyes.

The other students in the classroom giggled nervously, and waited patiently for Sam to begin reading. Then, the entire room hushed and silently waited. But, Sam was sure that he heard, no felt, Dorian giggling. It had to be Dorian. Sam thought he was blessed that way. He could feel and see things that other people could not see or feel. He felt Dorian giggling. It had to be him, and it could be no one else.

The silence was broken only when the whole class nervously giggled again, waiting for Sam to start reading. But, Sam wanted to laugh out loud. His eyes were closed. He could not block his ears. He wanted to read. He would, if he could have. It was Sam's turn to read out loud in class. It always ended this way and he wondered why he even needed to come to school. He did not learn anything and it was always a place for pain and for more tears. "Gasterre said I was dumb as a rock so why even bother coming to school?"

Sam asked himself. Sam wanted to be strong and show the entire class that he could be strong; therefore, he decided to start to read.

"One dark night, when…when…he…was in the woods…"

"Sam, if you cannot read the lesson, then sit down," Mrs. Gasterre snarled.

"One dark night, when he was in the woods, he saw a band of…a band of…"

"One dark night, when he was…"

"Sit down!" Gasterre finally said.

"Sit down," she said. Sam did as he was told and eagerly sat back down onto the hard backless bench. Sam sat wishing it were a stone. That way he could have melted into the raw stone and disappeared. His back was raw, stinging, and burning from the caning. This time he was glad that the benches did not have backs. His back was raw from the beating and he knew he would have yelled out in more pain from the back of any chair, or if Gasterre came anywhere near him.

Sam sat in the classroom facing the blackboard and Gasterre was standing towards the open door. He opened his eyes and looked her over. He looked at her face. Her skin was a perfectly unblemished caramel color. Her eyes were bright and deeply set. She was considered pretty even though her nose was slightly too big, though straight, but out of proportion to the fine facial features that she possessed. Her hair was black and closely cropped to her head. Her horn rim glasses were propped just above her eyebrows on her very large forehead. Otherwise, her head was perfectly round and her chin was shaped like a tear drop. Everyone thought she was pretty and she knew that everyone thought so. She stood erect, bold, upright, and confident in that knowledge.

Sam looked at her dress. The dress looked like a tent. The dress was shapeless, formless, and dull, but she cinched the waist in with a large orange-colored leather belt. The buckle was larger than the belt's width. If you were unfortunate to have the cane break during a beating, and she had to use that belt, God help you. She would make certain that the belt's buckle struck your back. The onslaught of the metal and the grating of the prong or tongue on your back were intolerable. The frame of the buckle was also decorated with jagged and uneven ornaments so that even that part created scars and scraped your back when it struck the skin. Gasterre's dress looked like one of the robes Esther, his mother, wore at home. Esther only wore a robe when she was doing house work. His mother would not wear anything like that out of the house, and certainly not to school. Esther was proud to say that she was a Gemini and that anything she put on, whether old or new, in-style or out-of-style looked great on her. Esther had been to the school too many times to count to meet with the several teachers and the school's principal concerning Sam's behavior. What was wrong with Sam? What was wrong with him? The calls were the same and the conversations were the same. Nothing ever changed.

Sam looked Gasterre up and down. What was wrong with Gasterre? Gasterre was short and well built. She was as tall as she was wide. Her arms were thick. Her fingers were long and supple. The knuckles were hardened and discolored. The cuticles lacked nail polish, were short, and closely cropped to the tips of the fingers. Those hands could as well have been the hands of a fighter or of a pianist. She used hers, not to create anything of beauty, but to inflict pain and misery, at least on Sam anyway.

Gasterre wore stockings that were tight and that matched her complexion. But through the stockings, Sam could see that her thighs were ample, her knees narrow, and her calves muscular. But, from the calf all the way down to her ankles, the definition and shape was completely lost. There was no tapering or narrowing of the leg at the ankle. Her legs were sturdy and they helped to hold up an even sturdier body. Someone had smiled in her favor and had given her a pretty face. And, someone must have found her somewhat attractive, at least at some point in her miserable life, for she wore a simple gold wedding band on her left fourth finger. Someone put a wedding ring on her finger and married her. Someone must have liked or even loved her. It was obvious however, that she did not like Sam. In fact he thought that she hated him. He must have triggered some deep place of disgust that he could not understand.

What was wrong with Gasterre? What had he ever done to her?

What was wrong with Sam?

…Ankles, smankles…That's what Gasterre walked on.

Crack, crack, crack…More licks rained down on Sam's back.

Life Force

Mr. Iguzi's ankles were not like 'smankles.' His ankles were much too thin. The right one was now broken, dangled, and deformed. The meaty flesh hung precipitously and the blood congealed at the open wound. The body was trying to heal itself and prevent its life force contained in the blood from wasting and spilling unnecessarily.

"Paloma, I think he needs more pain medication. Give him more now," I said. "And, oh, we need Ortho, STAT."

"Did you hear me? We need Ortho and an X-Ray STAT," I repeated, while I quickly put on a pair of sterile latex gloves. I felt that I was starting to chat too much and I knew that she had heard me the first time. I looked up while I was pulling on the gloves but Paloma was already gone. I turned away from the sink where I was standing and quickly checked Mr. Iguzi's pulses and the sensation in his feet. I cautiously replaced the skin that should have been covering the tibia. The skin would best serve as the natural protection to keep the leg from being exposed to the outside elements, dirt, and germs, any longer.

"Get Ortho, STAT," I repeated, "Mr. Iguzi needs to go to the operating room now." With this type of the injury we needed to get him to the operating room immediately. He needed to have the injury washed out and for the bone doctors to fix the ankle. The orthopedic surgeons would need to take off the dead tissue and put his ankle and foot back together. They would put nails, screws, and wire plates into his ankle.

The technicians from the radiology department responded quickly, and came into the room pushing the portable X-Ray machine. Mr. Iguzi appeared as if he still needed more pain medication. I decided to give more pain meds, before we had to move his leg, and to gingerly slide the X-Ray cassette under the bed's mattress. He was not on the usual trauma stretcher where the entire underside of the bed had a grooved area under the mattress to accommodate sliding in radiology film cassettes. With those trauma beds you do not have to move the patient at all. Other nurses and emergency room technicians came to help us, and we started to do the necessary work to get him ready to go to the operating room. They all worked in unison getting an EKG, drawing blood, and hanging up antibiotics. I also needed to get more of a history from him.

I took off the first pair of gloves that I was wearing. I washed my hands with soap and water, and put on non-sterile gloves this time to do the rest of the examination of the body. There did not seem to be any other areas of injury or open cuts, but I had to look all over him to be certain.

"Sir, do you want us to call someone for you?" I asked.

"Who knows that you are here? We need to let your family or someone know that you are here. How's the pain, on a scale from one to ten?"

"Still a ten," Mr. Iguzi said.

Paloma had already rushed back into the room carrying several vials of pain medications with her. I asked Paloma to give him more, and to give him a sufficient amount if needed to take the pain away.

I looked at his face to see if the pain was gone. I thought Mr. Iguzi was being a hero. He did not make a face. In fact, it was hard to read any emotion from just looking at him. With an injury like that I am sure you feel like jumping out of your skin. But the pain kept him from moving and without an expression. This was probably the calm before the storm. At any moment I expected Mr. Iguzi would grab my hand and scream out in pain. That reaction was common when you were in severe pain. You wanted to share it with someone. Holding on to someone or something helped to take the pain away. But, Mr. Iguzi lay there serenely as if connecting with a higher source of energy to cope with his pain.

I loved working with this team. They were focused and worked to get the job done. The members would know the next steps and speak out loud what they were doing. Doing that made it less confusing. We wanted to save Iguzi's ankle and foot. We wanted him to get back to do all the things that he liked—walking, jumping, skipping—whatever. If he went to rehab and did what the therapists asked, in no time he could be like "brand new."

<hr />

Sam chuckled and said that Gasterre had "ankles-smankles." He had confided to me that his teacher was ugly and that he hated her. But I had been to his school and I knew that she was not physically ugly. Esther had gone to the school many times because of some problem or other with Sam. Occasionally, I would go with her and sat in the car waiting while Esther went to the administration building to talk to the teachers. I had more than glimpsed Gasterre so I knew that she was not that bad looking. Usually Esther and Sam returned to the car and they would be quiet. Sam would sit quietly, emotionless, and would want to talk sometimes, but most times he would just be silent and clam up.

I always thought that Gasterre was not in equilibrium. Her face was certainly pretty but not in balance with the rest of her body. Her body was too thick and too muscular. Sam had said that Gasterre was mean. He had said that she had a mean streak and that it came out at the times when you least expected it. Sam wanted to know why she really had to be that way. It seemed that Sam was unfortunate to always bring out that mean streak in her. I guess he must have pushed some button. He was not her pet, nor was he any teacher's pet.

Sam hated that classroom. It was too bleak and there was hardly any light there. Gasterre had always kept the louvered windows closed. As other students and teachers walked by, Sam would crane his neck like a goose to see the shadows moving from the breaks in the louvered panes. He had no idea what was coming his way until – bam – it was right smack in front of him and they had stepped into the doorway. He did not like surprises.

There was only one door to the classroom. There was no sunlight streaming in, no natural lighting. Sam worried about being trapped in the classroom. What if there was a fire? How do we all get out of here?

"Sam," Gasterre said, "you would do as you always do. If you would only follow instructions and do as you were told you would not have so many problems. Raise your hand, wait to be called on, and I will tell you when to leave," Gasterre said.

Sam had no intention to wait for her. She would have looked at him over her wire rim glasses, snarled her lips, and only venom would come out. No, he would not wait for her to tell him to line up against the wall to leave the room, one by one. If there were to be a fire, Sam was sure that Gasterre would let everyone else leave before he did. He knew her well and knew what she would have done. Sam thought that she hated him so much that she would have probably blocked his way out with her ample body and left him in there to pass out, inhaling all the deadly smoke. She would have left him there to rot.

Gasterre did not allow finger paintings. None of the students could do that, and display their creativity and childlike fantasy on Gasterre's classroom wall. There was no macaroni art and no painting of Easter eggs. In fact, there were no paintings or art of any kind. She cared for a very bleak and dull wall.

...follow instructions and read the book...know the answer when called on, or else...crack, crack, crack...

"One dark night when he was in the woods...he saw a band of ... "

Mr. Iguzi's ankle was terribly broken. The bones were unbalanced and nothing about his leg was in equilibrium. The ankle and foot was out of balance. The foot dangled from its hinges. The spilled blood was thickened and blocked the port of exit from the wound. Mr. Iguzi smiled. It was unusual to see a smile from a patient in this situation. His leg was mangled, yet he was smiling. The smile was probably from a combination of finding a centering point for the pain and focusing on some unseen life force that reassured him that all would be okay. It could also have been from the repeated doses of pain medication that he had received. He was in a state of complete euphoria. I waved to him goodbye and good luck. The nurses and orthopedic surgeons did not even wait for me to say goodbye. They whisked him away on the stretcher to the operating room to get his ankle fixed.

"Goodbye and good luck," I whispered.

CHAPTER 2

SANDBURNED

I rubbed both eyes and blinked several times to adjust my contact lenses. I was not seeing too clearly and everything appeared blurry. It seemed that one of my contacts was stuck under my upper eyelid. I blinked again hoping that the contact would come down over my cornea, and sit correctly over my pupil to let me see clearly again. I reflexively reached up to touch my sclera, the white part of my eye, with my right index finger, to drag the contact back down onto its rightful place.

"Oh no. That is a no-no," I thought. My hands and fingers were certainly not clean. In fact they must have been filthy. I had been sitting on the bleachers eating a hotdog with ketchup and mustard and picking on greasy potato chips. I had now put all that mixture into my eye, the conglomeration of the condiments, bread crumbs, bacteria, viruses, fungus, and what-have-you.

Eventually, when I would start to work in the hospital, if the infection control nurse at the hospital had any inkling of that breach in protocol, or had seen me do that, it would have been a huge demerit in my record. After all, I had been well trained in universal precautions and knew to always use clean hand washing technique. I was so used to washing my hands before and after seeing each patient, before and after meals, and simply just washing my hands all the time. Cover your cough, sneeze into your armpit, and discard used tissue into a waste basket—by now you know the drill.

I would use the hand sanitizers that were everywhere in the hospital. How could you ever miss them? I wondered. The hand sanitizers were everywhere in rooms, hallways, cafeteria, on desks, everywhere. The ones on the portable stands jumped into you when you were walking around, distracted, aimless, and looking at your smart phone. They all said, "Healthy Hands Start Here." The hand sanitizers were everywhere: in malls, in restaurants, in offices, in supermarkets, and in gyms. For once I wanted to see a sign emblazoned with "Healthy Minds Start Here." That would be a great start for a call to action to reduce the stigma of mental illness.

I was extremely paranoid and fearful of putting germs into my eye and getting conjunctivitis. I did not want to walk around with my eyes blood shot red, infected, and unsightly looking. I did not want an eye infection, and could not bear wiping away the chunky yellow discharge that crusted at the upper and lower eyelids when you had an eye infection. If you were not careful to constantly wipe away the pus with a warm, clean, washcloth, you could easily rip away the eyelashes, and leave the borders of the lid barren and unsightly. I always only used the one-a-day contact lens and then tossed them away. I was fearful of having one red eye, or two red eyes. In fact, I was fairly paranoid about getting a bloody red eye or an eye infection. My fear bordered on a psychosis.

But that bully, Dorian, had thrown sand into Sam eyes when he was in the school yard. Sam had come home from school with both eyelids completely shut. Only a sliver of eyeball could be seen from them. And Sam had experienced such intense light sensitivity and pain that the paranoia about an eye injury was forever etched into my own brain.

———

It had all started because Sam had refused to give Dorian his lunch money that day. For whatever reason, Dorian's parents had not given him money to spend that day. Most likely they had, for Dorian's parents were professionals, or so he bragged daily to everyone. His father was an accountant and his mother was a nurse. Or she must have been a nurse at some time or another. She did not seem to work and I never saw her in a nurse's uniform.

"Give me your lunch money," Dorian said grinning. No one mistook the grinning as a joke. Dorian meant it as a command to Sam. It was not like Sam was going to have a choice that day. On previous occasions he had to give Dorian his money.

"Dorian, no, I can't," Sam replied.

"I only have enough to buy the milk powder and pay for the bulloh slush," Sam said. Bulloh slush was what we called the unrecognizable meat that the school served us at lunch time. You had no clue if it was chicken or beef or goat or pork or a combination of all of that. The only thing that you recognized was the watery, partially cooked, white rice that was served with the slush. Where was "Healthy, Hunger Free Kids" meals when you really needed it?

"Well, that's too bad," Dorian said.

"I need to get some candy," Dorian added. Dorian was a bully. He was very aggressive and he always seemed to get his way. He was the big boss of the school yard. On other matters he wasn't such a boss. He wasn't really smart but for whatever reason he always seemed to get fairly good grades. Sam was not paying too much attention to Dorian. But, he should have. Because out of the clear blue sky came a sand storm heading straight for Sam's face. Sam was not paying attention and he was not prepared.

Fluoush…

Sam's eyes intensely burned and his vision blurred. Sam could hardly see his own two hands. In fact, he could barely see at all. Instinctively, Sam dropped the coins that were in his hands, and he tried to cover his face and eyes. But it was too late. The small shiny coins fell to the ground. Quicker than quicksand and faster than a lightning bolt, Dorian grabbed them, darted, and ran. Smash and grab—that was the oldest of tricks.

Sam could not see and he squeezed his eyes shut. That, of course, made the burning worse. The pain was intense and the sand, gravel, and dirt in his eyes blocked his vision. Sam wanted to scratch his own eyes out. He needed to get the dirty sand out of his eyes. But, scratching and rubbing his eyes only made matters worse. The tiny particles of sand and dirt carved out train track marks all over his eyeballs. The white of Sam's eyes became blood shot red, and they roared alive with fire. The eye lids instantly became swollen and the lids closed in tightly. It was like the eyeballs were trapped in a Trojan horse; there was no further entry allowed, and there was no exit either.

Sam tried to open his eyes, but each time that he did, every grain grazed, and cut into the white sclera. It created little areas of bleeding on the eyeball. Satisfied with the damage to the white part of the eye that it had inflicted, the sand started to work on the cornea, and etched out grooves there. Why shouldn't it have? In its natural environment on a beach, that's what it did. It was meant to leave a trail, and create a pattern that anyone could see, discern, and follow.

Blindly, Sam made his way to the standing water pipe that was in the school yard. He gently fingered the pipe to find the top, and tried to turn the pipe on. His hands shook uncontrollably, and the intensity of the trembling, shaking, and fumbling delayed opening the top. Finally, the water came trickling down, and Sam made a cup of his hands to bring the water to his face. He was not working fast enough to get the pain to stop. In desperation, he finally put his head under the pipe. He hoped that would let the water flush the dirt, sand, and gravel from his face, and out of his eyes. It was a slow process, but the water took away most of the sand and dirt from his face. However, his eyes stilled burned.

Sam worked slowly, bit by bit, bit by bit, as his eyes tried to push the sand out of his eyes. But, the Trojan horse refused any of it to escape. The eyelids were too tightly shut. Sam worked slowly. He held his head under the pipe. While he was still holding his head under the pipe, the recess bell rang, and it was now time to return to the classroom. But Sam had resigned himself to having another day with no lunch. "Who cares, anyway?" he thought. It was bulloh, and it was slush. He hated to eat that food. You could never tell what meat it was.

Though the dirt and the sand on Sam's face were gone, his eyes were closed shut. He was not really hungry, and in any case, he didn't care. He would have nothing to eat. No bulloh. No slush. No milk. No lunch. Sam's eyes were bloody red and full of sand. He prayed that Gasterre would not ask him to read today. He knew that once she saw his swollen eyes, she would just assume that he was in a fight again. That was common. She would think that he had lost the fight and that he got punched in the eyes. Sam thought that Gasterre would have been happy to see that he got hit in both eyes. However, Gasterre was unusually kind today, and she did not ask Sam to read. Surprisingly, when she saw him like that she had asked if he was okay.

"Yes, Mam, I am okay," he said.

At the end of the school day, Sam waited for Esther to come to pick him up. Esther's heart raced when she saw him with his eyes looking like that. They were still tightly shut. Like everyone else, she assumed that he was in a fight, and got hit in the eye, both eyes. He was always in fights. What was wrong with Sam? Esther took one look at him, her heart raced, and she inhaled deeply. She held her tongue, and said nothing. However, undoubtedly, she knew that she had to take him immediately to the doctor to have his eyes examined.

Hold My Hands

It was almost as big as I was. Then again, I was never really that big in body. I was tall and lanky but not big. Our father had bought a water gun for Sam for his Christmas present. He had bought me a train set. This was one of the few Christmases that we had gotten any gifts. But, we loved those presents.

This was the only present that I had gotten that Christmas. I had played with the train set so much that soon several parts were missing. I took it out to the back yard and to the neighbor's house. I had lost the other parts very quickly and it had barely been a month. With the store bought toy broken we had to find some other way to entertain ourselves. We went back to making small nooses so that we could catch lizards. This was how we entertained ourselves in our spare time.

If not doing this, we would take parts of an old, used, garden hose and make a small wheel. We would get a wire hanger, straightening one end, and making the other end into the shape of a "U." We held it in our hands and drove the wheel around the yard and down the street. The best part of doing this was doing this in the rain. If you were really skillful you could steer the wheel through the rain water that was making its way down the street. The water would move rapidly along the side of the road and the sidewalk. If you could do this you really had a special skill with hand coordination and speed.

Sam did not play much with his water gun. He thought that his gift was something special. He was meticulous and finicky. He had taken good care of his present. I took care of mine too but, once mine was broken I needed some form of entertainment. Of course, Sam's toy water-gun was not getting much use. So why could I not use it? With repeated use and not taking good care of it, eventually, I broke Sam's toy. Sam was angry that I had broken his toy. He was so mad that I thought that I saw fire coming out the dragon's nose.

Sam was athletic and had a pretty good aim. He was snorting fireballs when he threw that vase at me. The green vase came at me from out of nowhere. He was aiming for my head. I had been standing by a tree that was in the back of the yard. I had taken a lemon from the refrigerator to eat as a snack as I loved to make the lemon slices zesty by sprinkling salt over each half of it. The extra tangy salt-lemon taste piqued the taste buds, and the mixture of the salt and lemon taste also brought on extra saliva into my mouth. You had to be careful to do this. If you were not careful pretty soon you would be drooling from the side of your mouth. The spittle made extra thin by the salt and lemony juices would flow as if it had found the rain leaders. And just like rain leaders that drain the water in the gutters from a house, if improperly placed, would allow the liquid to stay in one place, pooled and stagnant. That would leave a stain on your shirt if care was not taken to allow the liquid contents to drain and flow away properly. The lemon-salt taste heightened the senses. It stimulated the mind and it ignited the body. It was an energy booster. Like an adrenaline rush, that potion made you ready for anything.

I was lucky that my peripheral vision was good. I ducked just in time to miss the vase that would have slammed into my head. Swoosh. The green vase careened near my left ear. I had bent down just in time to avoid the vase colliding with the back of my head. With the force that he flung the vase I would certainly have been knocked unconscious by it.

"Ha, ha!" I laughed.

"Ha, ha!" I nervously giggled more. I was not sure what else he had up his sleeve. I should get ready. Should I fight or flee? Should I face the next missile or run? I nervously laughed and waited. I was calculating my options.

What should I do? If I fought him I would not win. I thought I was fast on my feet.

"Missed, missed…" I laughed.

I turned around and ran as fast as my spindly legs allowed. Everyone said that I had bird legs. I don't think that was meant to be a compliment. But these legs were good. These legs moved quickly and my bare feet grabbed the gravel and powdery earth and released them just as quickly. I ran away, not so much from fright, but in desperation.

I threw my body at the cast iron gates to fling them open. I barreled through the gates and ran down the street. I would have jumped over the gate to escape if I could have done so. I had seen Karl, Aunt Mitzie's husband, do that stunt when Lassie, our dog, had chased him in the yard. Lassie had every intention to rip the muscles in Karl's legs wide open. If Lassie had gotten hold of that calf muscle, the gastrocnemius and soleus muscles of his calves would have been torn to shreds.

Lassie had broken away from the leash that had kept her tied to the pipe stand. Once freed, Lassie had made one mad dash towards Karl. Karl did not appear to be any kind of athlete but, he gathered enough strength to hurdle the gate and he catapulted over the gate in one motion. He had been off and running down the street at full speed. Lassie stopped at the gate and laughed. Well, she appeared that she did. I imagined that the dog laughed and looked on in wonder on the meaty prize that got away so easily and gracefully.

Lassie sat down at the gate and wagged her tail, rolling her head from side to side in astonishment. "That one got away too easily. And he got away with such grace." I was not going to be so graceful. I knew that there was no way that I could get over the gate like that. Once I was at the gate I glanced back to see Sam now getting ready to run me down. I was faster on my feet and smarter and focused when in danger. So, just like Karl had done, I bolted down the street without looking back. At the end of Auburn Avenue and Duhaney Drive I had to stop to catch my breath.

All my breath was gone. I was breathless. I started to wheeze. I gasped for air. My chest was tight. I felt like I was drowning. I knew this must be what it felt like to be drowning. I wanted to get more air into my lungs. My asthma attack prevented all of that. No air would come in and none would go out.

Sam had broken my mother's green vase into three pieces. The base of the vase was intact. You could clearly identify it as the green vase. The vase knew its purpose was to be the container for a beautiful centerpiece display for flowers. It was meant to showcase those flowers, ferns, and leaves. The display would have brought joy to any home and party. Now the vase was shattered. However, despite that unexpected end, it was still recognizable as a vase. The base had a solid core and it could withstand any trauma, small or large. Sam was trying to kill me because I had touched his water-gun. Now, the water-gun was broken.

"Ha, ha, ha," I laughed.

"Missed," I said, "missed."

"You missed…missed, missed…"

"…missed, missed, ha, ha, missed…"

"Dr. Gary, we missed the vein in Room 18. We can't get the IV –intravenous line – in the patient in Room 18," Lise interrupted.

"All the nurses have tried but with no luck. The IV nurse from the floors tried, like five times, already. We can't even get a butterfly in so that we can draw the blood. All the veins are shot," she added. Lise was the emergency room nurse assigned to Rooms 17, 18, and 19.

"I have tried and tried. Nothing. You have to come do it and put a central line in," Lise said. She had already thought it through. She pushed the central line kit to me and waited for me to take it out of her hand.

"What size gloves do you take, eight or nine? I forgot."

"Everything is in the room for you. And make sure you get a red top, a blue top, and a purple top, just in case," she commanded. Lise had already read the patient's history. She had completed her examination of the patient and taken down the patient's reason for being in the emergency room. Based on that information she had figured out what blood work I might be ordering. She did not want to waste time once the central line was in place.

"Better get this over with, sooner than later," I said to myself.

I stood up pushing the chair back and away from me. I clicked out of the history of the patient that I was reviewing on the computer screen. I backed away from the workstation and put my pen in my lab-coat. I took the central line kit from her and said, "I take an eight, my gloves are eight."

Lise nodded and turned away to grab sterile gloves for me. I made a mental check of the other items I had to do when I came back to my desk. Go see the patients in Rooms 20 and 21. Call the cardiologist and the orthopedic surgeons who were on call today. Oh, the patient's family in Room 17 was still waiting for me to come to talk to them. They wanted an update on what was going on with their family member. I took a mental note—check, check, check, and check—and trying to keep all of that in my head. I was hoping that doing that mental check would make it easier for me to remember when I was finished with putting in the central line.

I walked into Room 18 and introduced myself to the patient. I showed him my name badge. I began by asking him what was wrong. Why was he here in the emergency room? I was taking his medical history and asking the questions as I stood at the side of the bed. When I was satisfied that I had gotten enough information, I said, "Mr. Wells, we need to put an IV in to get blood. We need to run some blood tests. The nurses were not able to get an IV in. So let me see what your veins look like."

I looked at his arms, forearms, hands, and neck. On both of his arms he had intricately designed tattooing. The design on his right arm was that of a knight slaying a dragon. The dragon looked angry, and fire was steaming out of its mouth and ears. The knight held a shield in his left hand, and a sword was raised in the right to smite the dragon. The body of the knight and the dragon were in dark blue. The snorted fire was in varying shades of red, orange, and yellow. On the left arm, the patient had a mermaid that looked longingly with forlorn eyes deeply at you. Her aqua scales exquisitely flowed downwards from the hips to splayed fins. The artist had painstakingly created an intricate design that made the mermaid look alive. It pulled you into it and caused you to stare at its otherworldly beauty. Mr. Wells must be used to people commenting on it, and it served as a start for a conversation.

"Wow, your tattoos are interesting," I said, going out on a limb.

"Did it take a long time to get those done? Did you do that in one sitting?" I asked.

I was making small talk while I was opening the central line kit. I unwrapped the packet with the size eight gloves, and opened the package for the gown that I was going to use.

"Oh, not a long time," he said.

"Oh, was it painful to get done?" I asked some more.

"Who came up with the designs, the art work?" I asked.

"Oh, I did. I like art. So, I researched the drawings for the knight, dragon, and mermaid. Finally, when I got to the ones that I liked, I took it to the tattoo parlor. I knew what colors I wanted and everything. It took me a couple of days. I had to go back several times to add the details that I wanted in them," he said.

"Wow," I said.

"So, who applied the tattoo?" I asked.

"Why do you ask?"

"Do you feel confident that they used good hygienic practices and always used a new needle on you?"

"What about the tattoo ink? Were these in singles bottles or multi-dose vials? Did they throw out the vials that the tattoo ink came in after they used them on you?"

"That tattoo ink is a great culture medium. That means that Hepatitis C grows very well in the tattoo ink. So every time they dip that needle into that ink, there is a risk for contamination. If the needle becomes contaminated with Hepatitis C, every beautiful tattoo mark they make on you puts you at risk of getting infected with Hepatitis C," I said.

"I am sure you made sure they used good, clean, universal precautions."

"You know, I am not so sure I even looked to see if they had a business license. Which I am sure they have one otherwise, they would not be open for business. On the other hand, I did not pay much attention to whether they used new needles and new bottles of inks," he replied.

"Well, not to get 'all up in your business,'" I said, even though I was already up in it.

"But, you know, there is a risk of getting Hepatitis C when you get a tattoo if unclean supplies are used," I said.

"Hepatitis C is a viral infection that attacks the liver. Once you get Hepatitis C, there is no cure."

"Oh, I did not know that."

"Yes, there is no cure. Some people who get Hepatitis C recover. But, a good portion of them do not recover and continue to have the virus in their blood and in their liver. If you are one of the unfortunate ones to whom this happens, the virus stays in your blood. With the continued presence of virus in your blood you can infect others with Hepatitis C. Hepatitis C can be transferred through sexual contact or through a blood transfusion that was infected with Hepatitis C. You can also get Hepatitis C through the sharing of needles and other items as toothbrushes. You cannot catch Hepatitis C by touching, shaking hands or standing next to someone. There are about 170 million people worldwide infected with Hepatitis C, also called Hep C for short."

"For some people, Hepatitis C causes a lot of damage to the liver. The liver may stop working and you get cirrhosis of the liver. With really bad cirrhosis of the liver, you can get really tired, fatigued, confused, and jaundiced. Jaundice means that your eyes become yellow. An infection with Hepatitis C can also put you at risk for getting liver cancer. If you get liver cancer or have cirrhosis you may need to get a new liver, that is, a liver transplant."

"Oh yeah? Is that right? I did not know that. I have heard some of my buddies talk about Hepatitis C, but did not really know what it meant. By the way, I don't share needles, if that's your next question," he said.

I smiled. That was my next question.

"Yes, that's good that you don't share needles," I said.

"There are many infections you can get with the sharing of needles. Of course, everyone knows about the risks of HIV if you share needles. But, there is also a risk of getting Hepatitis C if you share needles as well."

"I am glad that you do not share needles. That's a good idea not to share needles," I added.

"And, you know if you are going to get a tattoo, you should make certain that they only use new needles and new ink. Have them throw out the needles and all the ink when you are done."

"You may also want to know that the Centers for Disease Control, CDC, now recommend routine screening for Hepatitis C for all baby boomers, that is, those born between the years 1945 and 1965. The CDC estimates that the routine screening could save many lives by detecting the disease in the early stages and prevent some of the long term complications."

"If you are going to get a tattoo, you want to be sure that the persons giving the tattoos are properly trained and follow universal precautions. You want to be sure that they always use clean and sterile needles that have not been used on anyone else. Make sure they use gloves and open all the products in front of you so that you can see what they are doing," I said.

"Yeah, I wish I had known that before I got all these tattoos. I am done with my tattoos anyway, I don't need no more."

"Well, hey. Knowledge is power. I am sure you have many friends. You know what they say, each one, teach one," I said.

"Now that you know, you can tell your buddies about the risk of Hepatitis C with tattooing if clean supplies are not used. And, of course there is also the risk of HIV with sharing needles," I added.

"Well, let me see what we can do with finding a vein for this IV, this intravenous line."

Through the tattoos, I could see that most of the veins on the upper extremities were sclerosed, scarred down, hardened, and completely shot. He had used them all up. The dark blue knight and dragon hid the veins and it was hard to tell where a vein started and where one ended. The nurses in their attempts to get to the veins had stuck him too many times. There were folded two-by-two gauzes crisscrossed with tape to cover up were the nurses in their prior attempts had tried and failed. Similarly, on his left arm the mermaid had been jabbed and pricked by several needles. I knew I would be in trouble, for if they could not get the IV in, there was no use for me even trying his arms, as the nurses were the experts.

I said to him, "You know what, let me finish fully examining you first and then I will try to put a central intravenous line, IV, in." I was trying to strategize and optimize my time for the best course of action to save us some time.

He nodded and said, "Doc, I can tell you don't even bother wasting your time with looking at my arms. As you can see the tattoos make it hard to see the veins anyway."

"And, to be honest with you, Doc, I shoot drugs. I know where my best veins are. Most of them are done for. I told the nurse where the last one was but she could not get the IV in. And, I don't want you to place the IV in my neck. So do us all a favor and just put it in my thigh. They had to do that like the time before last," he added.

I nodded in agreement, appreciative that he would be so cooperative with placing the line in the femoral vein in his groin. I was not going to argue with that. It would make my life so much less complicated tonight. Less complicated is always good.

I also hope that he would tell his buddies about the risks with Hepatitis C with getting a tattoo, and the risk of HIV with sharing needles. We have enough problems already. "Why add insult to injury?" I thought.

I finished examining him, masked, gloved up, and put on the sterile garb in preparation to put the line in.

…missed, missed…

I tried to get the intricate tattoos out of mind. I tried to focus. I had to concentrate on the task on hand so as not to miss the vein on the first attempt. I had to hold my hands firm and prevent them from shaking. With most things in life, and certainly in the emergency room, time was of the essence. I had to focus, concentrate, be methodical, and hold my hands steady. Time was of the essence, but being distracted was also a problem. To have a complication while placing the intravenous line in his groin would not be a good thing at all

CHAPTER 3

THE SCENT OF LILAC

I t was eight o'clock in the morning and I was getting ready to take Sam back to the assisted living center. He must have had a restful night as he had not gotten up at all. Sometimes at night when he could not sleep he would get up and pace in his room. Invariably, after he had become tired of wearing out the tracks in his bedroom, he would come out into the hallway. He would go down the stairs and then start to pace in the kitchen. I was glad that did not happen last night. I had heard him snoring throughout the night. The muffled mouth breathing had come directly through my bedroom walls into my room. Because of the noise I had barely slept. Even with minimal sleep it was still time to start a new day. I went into his room and tried to wake him up so that he could take a shower.

"Sam, Sam, get up," I said.

Sam had sobered up a lot from the night before. Once awake, he sat up and flung his legs over the side of the bed. However, he did not move.

"Sam," I said, "you have to get moving because I need to be at work at 2 p.m. today. Let's get you in the shower now." I pulled on his left arm to help him up. I needed him to get into the shower right away. He rose slowly. I walked behind him to encourage him to go into the bathroom. Once there, I pulled the shower curtain closed. I turned on the bath faucet to get the water to a comfortable temperature. Once the temperature was adequate, I turned on the shower and ran it for a couple of minutes. Sam still stood there looking at me as if he did not know what to do.

"Sam," I said, "Take your clothes off and get into the shower." He slowly removed all of his clothing. I looked at him and contorted my face to express urgency. My cell phone started to ring. I looked down and saw that it was Brice. It was poor timing and I decided not to answer the phone right then. I looked back at the phone in my hand wondering what was up with Brice. I silently mouthed the words to Sam, "Let's go," and he reluctantly stepped into the shower.

Sam was not in the shower for more than a minute when he said to me, "Is this enough, have I bathed enough?"

"Sam," I said, "did you even use soap? You have to use the soap. Now, take the washcloth, put soap on it, and bathe. You need to get the soap all over your body, everywhere, including your back."

"Can you help me do it?" Sam asked.

"No, no, no," I said. "You know how to take a shower and bathe. I'm not gonna help you do it. You can do that by yourself. You can do that alone. I don't have to help you do that. Your hands and fingers and arms and feet still work. Nothing is wrong with them as far as I can tell."

Sam wanted to waste time in the shower. He could be obstinate. I stood my ground and decided not to help this time. I twirled the phone in my hand and stood there waiting for him to be done in the shower.

My cell phone rang for a second time. Again, it was Brice. He was calling a second time in less than a minute. "What does he want now so early in the morning," I said. "Sam, get out of the shower now," I said. "It's time to go."

I was thinking of all the things I had to get done before starting work at 2 p.m.

"Sam, look, let's get you back to the assisted living center. Charlie and Marlon can take over and help with getting you settled back in there. They can drive you over to the mental health center today. I will call Heather later and tell her what had happened," I said. I was sure Heather would have helped. Heather had been Sam's clinician for more than ten years. She had been an excellent source of help and support. I could not imagine doing all this work with Sam without her assistance. I was certain that they had not told Heather about what happened with Sam not getting to the center yesterday. Once she found out I was sure that she would not be a happy camper either.

I had laid out clean clothes for Sam on the bed and I told him to go get them on.

"You have to help me get my socks and sneakers on," Sam said. I nodded in agreement without saying anything more.

"Yeah, get your pants and shirt on. Then we can do the rest together," I said.

Sam sat on the bed and pulled on his shirt. He stood up to put on his pants. Once he got the pants on, he sat down heavily on the bed. I then bent down at the bedside to put the socks on. His ankles and calves were very swollen. They had probably gotten that way from him walking around and standing up all day yesterday. I thought that they must have been hurting. But, in his drunken state yesterday, he probably did not feel anything. His legs and feet must have gone numb from the stretching of the nerves and all the tissues in his leg.

"Lift your foot up so that I can get the socks on," I said. I had just put on the second sock when my cell phone rang for the third time. "Sam, come downstairs like that and I will put your sneakers on down there," I said. The call was from Brice again. He had not left a message the last two times. Now this was the third call. "This must be important," I said to myself. I was very tempted to ignore it for the third time, but this time I answered the call.

"Hello, Brice," I said.

"What's up, doc?"

"You tell me."

"I have a question for you."

"Please, go ahead."

"You can't return a call?" he said. "I called you, like three times, already this morning. Why did you not pick up? In fact, I called you more than five times yesterday and you didn't return my call. What's up with you? You can't return a call? Don't tell me that you're that busy that you can't return a call," he said.

"So is that why you called me? To ask me why I didn't return your call?" I asked. I chose to ignore his question and accusation about me being too busy to return a call. As far as I knew he had not become an investigative reporter. Therefore, I felt no need to detail my business, or lack thereof. What does my not returning a call have to do with anything about what was going on in my life? He should have just left me a message.

"Brice. You said you had a question for me? What is it?"

"Well, you know that I had prostatitis last year? Remember?"

"Yes. I remember."

"And, remember that Dr. Westphal gave me an antibiotic because the prostatitis did not go away with the first course of treatment. Remember?"

"Uhm, uhm. Yes," I responded half-heartedly.

"Well, now I am feeling that it's back again."

"Okay? So?"

"Well, my PSA was normal last year. Now I am feeling that this prostatitis thing is back."

"So are you saying that you feel the return of the prostatitis has something to do with your PSA?"

"Something does not feel right."

Brice worked out at the gym practically every day. I don't even know where he found all that time to do all that training. He did weight training and running. He also rode the stationary bicycle and did the treadmill. He was in excellent physical shape. He could bench press over three hundred pounds. That was considerably more than his weight. He was in better shape than many men half his age. "What was he so concerned about?" I wondered.

"Something's wrong. I know it. I went to Dr. Westphal and he told me that my PSA was higher," he said.

"Why did he check it again? You just had that done, what, less than a year ago?"

"I told him to do it."

I had been standing at the foot of the stairs on the first floor waiting for Sam to come down. The telephone's reception was much better from this point in the house anyway. I was trying to listen to Brice and watch Sam come slowly down the steps. I stood there watching Sam come down the steps. It was probably a mistake to have him come down the steps with only socks on. That increased the likelihood of him falling. Brice's telephone call had distracted me and I was not paying attention to safety details. Sam was not using his cane as he should have and he really needed the cane to keep his balance. Usually, I would have held the cane and helped Sam come down the steps. Once he was on firm landing I would give the cane back to Sam. Since he had already come down the stairs without the cane I sighed with relief. He had come down without incident. "Sam. Sit on the sofa. I will be there in a second to put your sneakers on," I said.

"What about sneakers?" Brice asked.

"Not you, Brice, not you," I said. I had not moved the cell phone from my lips when I started to talk to Sam. I had not told Brice to hold on so that he would know that conversation was not meant for him.

"Brice, are you thinking that you have prostate cancer?" I asked.

"Yes, my PSA went up. I don't want to get cancer," Brice said.

"My father had colon cancer. I watched him die slowly. I watched him in pain. I don't think that I can deal with that kind of pain," he said.

"Brice," I said, "the way medicine is practiced today has changed so much since your father's time. The treatments available then, and those available now are so different. What your father went through at that point in time is most likely not the same if he had that same problem today," I said.

"Besides, if you are thinking about prostate cancer, I doubt that you have that. The numbers that you just told me are really the same number. Your PSA is normal," I repeated. Brice liked to have information repeated more than once. He would latch onto an idea and not budge from it. He was extremely intelligent and I think this was how he memorized information. His recall was excellent. If you had a question about some historical event, in a split second, he would give you the answer. But, I know that I also frustrated him by asking too many questions, and not always answering my phone. He helped me to understand that different people take in information in different ways and at a different pace. He helped me to become much more patient than I inherently was.

"Yes, but something is wrong. I am so scared to get prostate cancer," Brice said.

"Well, Brice. Nobody wants cancer. Nobody wants a physical illness. Nobody wants a mental illness either," I said. "But sometimes things happen. Some things are under our control and some things are not. But what we should be doing is finding a way to deal with the problem. When we face a problem squarely it is an opportunity to find a solution." I said. "As we learn more, we know that prevention is better than the cure. Let's prevent the problem in the first place."

"So, Brice, did you tell Dr. Westphal that you had other symptoms? Was something else wrong?"

"No," he said.

"Well, do you have problems when you first start to pee, starting the stream?" I asked.

"No."

"When you pee is the flow weak, or stops and starts again?"

"No."

"Are you peeing a lot, especially at night?"

"No, I don't have that either. But, what's wrong with me then?" he asked, interrupting my string of questions.

"I hear you," I said.

"Do you mind if I ask you a couple more questions?"

"Do you find it hard to empty your bladder completely? Or feeling that it is not empty?" I asked.

"Have you had any pain or burning during peeing, seeing blood in the pee or semen, any pain in your back, hips, or pelvis that won't go away?"

"No. I don't have any of that either," he said.

I knew that sometimes men don't feel anything or have no symptoms at all with prostate cancer.

"From what you have just told me your PSA is normal. You have no symptoms whatsoever," I said.

"Well, Bob, my friend just told me he did not have any problems. Then he went to the doctor and they found out that he had prostate cancer," Brice countered. He wanted to point out that having no symptoms might not make a difference.

"True," I said, "different men have different symptoms. Some men do not have any symptoms at all. Yeah. I would not use Bob as an example."

"First, he may not tell you everything that he is going through. You are not his doctor. You are not his confidant. Who really knows what he was feeling or going through."

"And, when was the last time he went to a doctor anyway?" I asked. "It is a good idea to have regular checkups with your health care provider. When you go regularly, your health care provider can do the necessary screenings. They can do the preventive testing or treatments that you need. You should not wait until you feel sick."

"When you go regularly, the provider can catch the problems. It is better to find out the problem in its early stage. Preventing the problems in the first place is even better," I added.

"I go to the doctor all the time," Brice said.

"I know you do. You have all your prevention screens done. Anyway, Brice, your PSA is normal. And, you told me that you had a prostate ultrasound last year. That was normal."

"You had a full workup last year with blood work, more tests and scans," I said.

"I am just anxious I guess because of what Bob told me."

"Sure, it is natural for uncertainty to bring on some anxiety."

"I think your numbers say that you are fine and you are in good health."

"In any case, your best bet is to have Dr. Westphal examine you once more," I said.

"Doc, you know I take pills for anxiety, right?" Brice asked.

"Yes, you did tell me that you have an anxiety disorder. Brice, that is cool with me. Even *Iron Man* had anxiety and panic attacks."

"I took a pill this morning because I was getting myself all worked up."

"I think you did the right thing."

"Are you still seeing your doctor and going to the therapist regularly?"

"Keep the appointment with Dr. Westphal, Okay?" I said.

"Yeah, yeah, you know I will."

"So what are you up to so early this morning?" Brice asked.

"Oh, don't ask," I thought, but did not say.

"Well, I have Sam with me," I said. "And, I have to get him back to assisted living before I have to go to work for 2 p.m."

I had gotten so caught up in the conversation with Brice that I had forgotten that Sam was still waiting for me to come to put his sneakers on.

"Brice, look, I got to run."

"Do you have any other questions for me?" I asked.

"No. Look, I will call you later and tell you what Dr. Westphal said."

"Good. My cell phone is on. Call when you can. But, don't forget that we are to go to the football game on Sunday."

"Okay, later." I disconnected from the call and went over to the sofa to help Sam put his sneakers on. I had to get him back to the assisted living center.

"One thing at a time, one thing at a time," I said to calm myself so that I would not become too overwhelmed by all the tasks at hand today.

By 2 p.m. I was at work and I had a medical student to work with me.

"Connor, please go to see the patient in Room 8 first and then tell me what you think," I said.

Connor was a fourth year medical student doing a rotation in the Emergency Department. He was shadowing me today. He had already gone through the clinical diagnosis classes and knew how to examine patients. This was not his first clinical rotation. He had done all the core rotations during the third year of medical school. He had done rotations in medicine, pediatrics, general surgery and psychiatry. He had also done electives in orthopedic surgery, anesthesia, and ear, nose and throat surgery already. Therefore, in the fourth and his final year of medical school, he should know what he was doing.

He should be able to review the complaints and symptoms, examine the patient and come to an assessment of what was the most likely diagnosis. He should also be good at making a short list of diagnoses. That means considering what other diagnoses were possible given what he found out by talking to and examining the patient, any other clues he found and reviewing any additional supporting information. At this stage he should be good at putting it all together. He should be able to come and tell me what other tests, labs, X-Rays, or scans we would need to do to get to the correct diagnosis.

"You want me to see the patient first without you?" Connor asked.

"Yes," I said. "You may go first and then tell me what you think."

"Come back with three possible diagnoses, tops. Nothing more, nothing less."

Being in the emergency room as a young medical student can be nerve wracking. Everything happened too fast. The patient could be sitting up in the bed telling you about the chest pain that she was having. You would be signaling to the nurse or tech to come in to the room to obtain a 12-lead EKG. You would know that something was not right because her heart rate was high and the electrical tracing on the monitor was erratic. But, in the twinkling of less than an eye the patient who was talking to you could clutch her chest, collapse on the bed, and code right in front of you. In that split second, the world around you crashed and tumbled to a standstill.

Any patient could have sudden cardiac death without warning. We would all dash to the room with the crash cart. You would thump the chest —one, two, three thumps. You would shock and defibrillate the heart to try to resuscitate the patient. Everything changes. The status of people could change rapidly in the emergency room. If you were a person who did not like to live with change the emergency department was not a good place to work. It was unpredictable and changing. Anything could come crashing through the room doors. Unpredictable.

Connor went off to Room 8 to examine the patient. He came back too soon. So, I looked up at him. I knew that he could not have reviewed the nurse's notes and found out so quickly why the person was in the emergency room. He certainly had not examined the patient in that space of time. He would also need to take a minute or two to put it all together, think about the most likely diagnosis, and come back to me.

So, what was up? What about more tests? He certainly did not already think about all of that? If more testing was needed, what were they? The patient must be really sick for him to come back so soon.

"Dr. Gary, I think you better come right away," Connor said.

"Why?"

"Well, I read through the triage nurse's notes. You know, the notes that the first nurse out in the waiting room writes when the patient comes into the emergency room. She is the one who takes down the complaints from the patients."

I smiled. I am quite familiar with the concept of triage. Connor was getting nervous and telling me the obvious.

"Yes, Connor, I know about the triage nurse and their notes."

"Sybil, the nurse working in the room, told me I should come to get you now. She was in the room examining the patient when I walked in. She told me to come get you at once."

"She was putting oxygen on the patient. Then she listened to his heart and lungs. Sybil started to listen to the abdomen with her stethoscope. She looked up at me and told me to come get you. Sybil said she thinks the person as an aneurysm."

"Aneurysm? Where? In the head, chest, or belly? Where is it?" I asked.

We started to walk quickly and almost ran to Room 8.

"Why is the patient in the emergency room today?" I asked. "Was it a headache, chest pain or belly pain?"

"The patient had complained of back pain. The pain went down his back and into his thighs."

"How old is he?"

"He is sixty seven. He had also some abdominal pain, but that went away."

"So he had back and belly pains? What's the blood pressure and pulse?" I asked. Connor gave me the numbers for the blood pressure and the heart rate.

"Did you get a chance to see what other medical problems he has? Has he had any surgeries, takes any medications, or have any allergies? Does he still have chest pain? Are you sure the abdominal pain is gone? Does he have risk factors, like high blood pressure, high cholesterol, and smoking? Did you check the pulses in all the extremities? Did you check his pulse in the thigh at the femoral artery and pulses elsewhere? How many intravenous lines did Sybil place in him? Did she already do an EKG and get him typed and crossed? Is there any family with him?" I asked all the questions in rapid succession. I had not given Connor any chance to answer any of the questions. My thoughts had revved and I was thinking ahead about the possibilities. But, I reminded myself not to jump to conclusions. Ask the questions, examine the patient, and put all the pieces of information together to get to the correct answer.

"No, I did not get a chance to ask him any of that," Connor said.

"I came to get you at once. Sybil said I should come get you to come at once."

"Absolutely, that's fine," I said smiling. I smiled to reassure Connor that he had done the right thing by coming to get me as Sybil had asked.

In less than ten seconds we were in Room 8. The patient was awake and talking, but he seemed a bit anxious. I looked at the vital sign monitor mounted over the bed. The patient was breathing comfortably on oxygen. Sybil had put on him a nasal cannula to give him more oxygen and the tube's prongs were propped in his nose. Sybil had secured the tubing by looping it over his ears. I took a mental photo of the contours of his neck and jaw. His neck was thin and long and his jaw was sturdy and protuberant. The distance from the angle of the jaw to the tip of his chin was adequate. It was not shortened and it did not abruptly end. When he spoke to answer Sybil I saw that he could open his mouth wide enough. "Good, that's a plus for him and me if we need to intubate him and put a tube in his throat," I thought. The tube would connect him to the breathing machine.

The blood pressure was a little better than what it had been less than a minute before. The monitor's screen was alive with four separate tracings displayed in various colors. The lines kept on moving, tracing out different patterns based on what it was measuring. The patterns were repetitive and the alarms were silent. There was no ding, ding, dings, or the sputtering noise of paper printing because the numbers were outside the normal ranges.

"Okay, well let's see what we have here," I said.

Mr. Allen was lying on the bed trying not to pay too much attention to Sybil. She was slapping and flicking on the veins on his left arm to make the veins stand out, and trying to make the veins pump up with blood. This would make it easier to place a second intravenous line.

"Ah, good," I thought.

Sybil and I were thinking along the same lines. Sybil had already placed one large bore IV in the right arm. She was now teasing the veins of the left arm. It was important for him to have a second line.

"I know you will need these," she said. "In fact, I knew that you were going to tell me to put in two large bore IVs and draw more blood work. I am one step ahead of you."

"Well, you must have been," I mumbled. Yes, you must have been. Connor already told me you thought the patient had an aneurysm. How could she know? Did she do all the tests to confirm her suspicions?

"Was she prescient? Could she see into the future?" I wondered. Some people claimed they could see into the future. I was not one of them. I did not claim that I could nor did I claim that I would at some point.

Sybil seemed to be getting the patient ready to go the operating room. I was thinking about the possible complications of an aortic aneurysm and the risks of surgery. The aneurysm could dissect and rupture. The dissection could lead to poor blood supply to the lower body and to the spinal cord. This could result in paraplegia, weakness, and loss of muscle function in the lower legs. The patient's blood pressure could become unpredictable with an aneurysm. It could get high then rapidly get low. That could put the patient at risk of having a stroke or a heart attack. The stress on the heart could also bring on an irregular heart rate. That abnormal rhythm of the heart could result in death. Why did I want to go down that line of thought, anyway? That was like crossing the bridge before you even got there. Or like forcing a horse to drink at a river that did not exist before you even led the horse to the river. What did they call that? Soothsaying? Was this a premonition or just plain old negative thinking? Was that kind of negative thinking ever useful? Not really. I tried to think only with positive thoughts.

But positive or negative let's find out what is wrong first. First, let's get to the correct diagnosis. We had to be sure that the diagnosis was correct. I know that we needed some type of image, radiology, to confirm that indeed there was an abdominal aortic aneurysm. I let Sybil continue to do her work. I introduced myself to the patient and I began to ask the same questions again. Mr. Allen looked at me and said, "I just told the nurses that. It's the same questions and the same answers," he said.

"Oh, yes, I know that you have done that," I said.

"It is really important for me to ask again to be sure that we have the story right. Sometimes when we ask the same thing over and over, you remember a detail, something that you had forgotten to tell us," I said.

I glanced up at the vital signs again to make sure that they were good. I asked all my questions again and got the same answers as the others had.

"Okay, are you in pain now?" I asked.

"No," Mr. Allen said.

Mr. Allen repeated his story about what had been happening to him over the last month. He was sixty seven years old and had high blood pressure and high cholesterol. He was a smoker. The mid back and abdominal pain started over a month ago. At first, the pain was only in his back, it started to go into his buttocks and groin. Eventually, the pain in the buttocks and groin stopped. Now he only had some mild back pain. He had only come to the emergency room because he wanted to make sure that it was "nothing." His blood pressure had been high but he had stopped taking the medications. "Forget about cholesterol," he said. He did not want to take that medicine for it. In fact, he had also stopped going to his primary care provider for over a year now. He said that he felt fine so he did not see the need to go. I always hated to say "I told you so," but that decision was probably not a good one. I supposed that if he had gone, his doctor would have recommended a screening. Given the risks that he described he may have had an ultrasound to look for the presence of an aneurysm. Listening to his story and examining him, that is what I thought he had. I thought he had an abdominal aortic aneurysm. Based on the risk factors of his age, high blood pressure, high cholesterol, and smoking, I think his doctor would have sent him for an abdominal ultrasound. Now he was in the emergency room with an emergency condition. It probably did not have to happen that way. One cannot predict the future, but prevention certainly would've been better than cure.

I think that Sybil and Connor were both correct. On physical examination Mr. Allen had a bruit, a noise or muffled sound. He had a bruit that was obvious when you listened over the aorta in his mid-abdomen. There was no pulsatile mass to suggest that the aorta was getting bigger as we speak, rupturing or dissecting. We planned to get all his blood work drawn and to do a CAT scan of his abdomen. We needed to find out what was going on with his aorta. If indeed he had an aneurysm we needed to know how big it was. I grabbed the hospital's mobile phone out of my lab-coat pocket.

"David, hey, what's up? Do you have anyone on the CAT scan table now?" I asked. David was the CAT scan technician. He was one of the best CAT scan technicians. He was responsive, courteous, and professional.

"I have a patient, Mr. Allen, in Room 8. We need a CAT scan of his abdomen and pelvis, STAT. We need to look at the aorta," I said.

"Are you looking for an aneurysm?" David asked.

"Yes, David, we think he has an abdominal aortic aneurysm," I said.

"Do the cuts through his chest as well. So, we need the CAT scan angiogram study of the chest, abdomen, and pelvis. He is stable. But, we need to see what the aorta looks like," I said.

"Sybil will bring him up on the monitor," I said.

"Do you have the creatinine?" David asked. "We don't want to knock out his kidneys. The load of dye that he will get with the CAT scan angiogram may do so even though it is not a lot."

"Of course," I responded. "We just got the creatinine back from the lab."

"His creatinine is normal," I said. "His kidneys work."

"I will call and tell the vascular surgeons that we are doing the CAT scan to look for an aneurysm," I said.

I would hate to call them to say that we have a patient with a large or rupturing aneurysm on the CAT scan table and not to have given them any warning. We needed to warn them. People say they like surprises but I did not find that to be the case. Only birthday surprises are fun, I thought. The other surprises, well, it depends. Let's get all our ducks in a row," I said. "Let's not surprise them that way."

"David, as soon as it is done, let the radiologist know. Call me, okay? We don't have time to lose," I said.

Events change. People change. The status of people could change rapidly in the emergency room. Mr. Allen was stable and the aneurysm was not dissecting or rupturing. If the blood pressure fell and he was in a shock state we were prepared. Preparation was the key. Sybil had placed two large bore IV lines in his arms. All the blood work was drawn and had been sent to the lab. The EKG was normal. I had taken a mental note of Mr. Allen's neck, throat, and jaw. If anything unexpected happen I was sure that I could manage his airway I would have been able to easily put an endotracheal tube into his airway. In the emergency room you always went back to the basics.

You focused on the core principles. Know your ABCs. You always made sure that you secured the airway. You needed to get oxygen to the patient by any means. B was for blood pressure. You had to make sure the blood pressure was somewhere near normal. C was for circulation. You had to make sure that the oxygen and the blood got to the vital organs: the brain, the heart, the lungs, and the kidneys. The oxygenated blood had to get to all the tissues and muscles. If you did not start with the basics, all the other heroics would be for nothing. Know your ABCs. If you mastered the core principles and went back to the basics you should be able to withstand any change. When the unexpected and unpredicted happened, and they always do, you can be better prepared and easier adapt.

The last time that we had an aortic aneurysm rupture right before our eyes in the emergency room, the patient had come in with back and abdominal pain and in less than a minute, he was a Code Blue. That had not been a successful resuscitation. But this was not going to be the case today. Sybil, with her foresight, had him already in the operating room. I crossed my fingers. I would have crossed my toes too except that they were in socks and shoes. For good luck, I wanted the CAT scan to come back to say that he had an aneurysm but that it was not so large, or dissecting, and that he did not need to go to the operating room today.

However, with the memory of that disaster floating back into my consciousness, I instinctively held my breath to suppress it. I was still holding my breath but told myself to remember to breathe.

Breathe, breathe.

Otherwise, I would suffocate.

Sybil was prescient. She probably thought she had foresight. She was seeing way beyond the diagnosis and into the operating room. The diagnosis I was certain was correct. But her premonition about what would happen in the operating room, today of all days I wanted her to be so wrong.

I was still suffocating. I could not breathe. I felt I was choking. My chest was tight. An elephant sat on it. I could not move my limbs. The scent of lilac was everywhere. I was on the verge of having an asthma attack. I was in a phase of sleep paralysis or apoplexy. This usually happens at the transition between falling asleep or waking up. I was not asleep in a strange bed. Sleep paralysis was more likely to happen when sleeping in unfamiliar surroundings.

Who had been spraying that smell around? The scent was everywhere and it was seeping into everything. It seeped through my nostrils and found its way into my lungs. It permeated my clothes and saturated my skin.

I sat in the second row of seats in the church. My skinny body hardly took up much of the bench. I leaned all the way back and half my legs still dangled in mid-air. I did not want to lean forward. If I had done that, leaned forward, my back would not be supported by anything. It was not a comfortable bench for me or anyone else to sit on.

They came in slowly, one by one. They stopped and took Maman's and Miss Iris's hands into their own hands, shook and quickly released them. It was the same reaction when you told people about mental illness in your family or in yourself. They would apologize as if it were their fault. They felt your pain, and quietly said so. They would shake your hand, but at the end of the handshake you felt them subtly pushing you away. It was too close for comfort.

The mourners leaned forward and whispered something into Maman's and Iris's ears. I could not hear what they said. No one could. Maman's and Iris's eyes glazed over. But at some point, I thought that I could make out that they were saying, "Thank you. Thanks for coming."

Their eyes were filled with tears. At any moment now, the gobs of tears would just brim over, and sliver down their cheeks. I could see that the handkerchiefs they held were already soaked. People kept on streaming in one by one, single file. They looked appropriately pious, cast their eyes downwards, shook their hands, and kissed their cheeks. They whispered in their ears but moved away from the family too quickly.

Mr. John Blue was there as he seemed to be everywhere these days. His usual too tight dark blue pants were made of polyester and he hiked them up all the way over his belly. I thought he invented the color blue as everything he wore was blue. Blue. He wore a blue jacket and a blue shirt. The ensemble was complemented by a blue tie. I was certain that at one point the shirt had been white. But now it too was blue. I looked at his shoes and they were blue too. Where does a man get blue shoes to buy? John Blue had made his fashion statement. Mr. Blue must also have been the weather man and he predicted that a flood was coming soon. His pants were too short, and his ankles and socks were showing. When the flood finally came, only he and his ankles would be dry and safe from the deluge.

Where was Mrs. Blue, anyway? I wondered. Maybe there was not one. Most likely he didn't have a mirror either. He had no wife, no companion, no significant other or lover, no friends, and no mirror. That's must be why he was everywhere. No human contact and no mirror, no one to give him feedback. That was a recipe for disaster and a set up to be in public looking wrong. That would be the case when you have no one to reflect with or to keep you in check. You would have no one to tell you to change that pants or that tie. No, you cannot wear this with that. That tie did not go with that shirt. He had nothing to help him to reflect.

I could not breathe. My lungs were tight. I could not see. I was choosing not to breathe. I chose not to see. The whiff of lilac percolated in my lungs. I was seated in the second row of the benches in the church. The coffin was too close to me. I could see. I did not want to see. I did not want to see anything. Miss Ivy had been the best neighbor, ever. But, one day she was there, and the next she was gone.

Esther, my mother, had taken Miss Ivy to the hospital as she had not been feeling well. Esther had said that Miss Ivy was sick and she had to go to hospital. By the next day, Miss Ivy was gone.

"Gone where?" I asked.

"Gone to heaven," Esther said.

"You mean died and gone to heaven?" I asked.

"Yes, died and gone to heaven," Esther said.

"Why?" I asked. Where was heaven? I asked. I still did not understand what Esther was saying.

"Why what?" Esther asked. She did not know what I did not get.

"Why did she go to heaven?" I asked.

"Miss Ivy was very sick. She was older and she was sick. It was her time and she was called home," Esther said.

"Oh. Am I gonna be called home too?" I asked.

"No. No. You are not going to be called home," Esther answered.

"That's good," I said.

Still, the coffin was much too close to me. I tried not to look at it.

Eventually, the church service started and everyone sat down. Their eyes were filling with tears. Once the service started several people got up to read and reminisce about Miss Ivy. The choirs sang and, despite the loud singing and mixture of voices, you could still distinctly hear Ms. Iris's soprano. She sang well and reached into the high vocal ranges. The sound of her voice permeated into my bones, touching my mind, body, and soul. The voice stirred my emotions as she sang and I was moved. Every soul was touched. Our bodies quivered and our minds were overcome with emotions. We were just on the verge of openly sobbing when the pastor came up to give his sermon.

"Yes, you are earth, dirt, ashes," he bellowed.

I could not listen to him as I was distracted by the smell of lilac. I could not see in front of me. I did want to listen. I could not. I did not want to look forwards. I did not want to look backwards.

A whiff of lilac came and the scent of lilac oppressed me. The first smell of lilac triggers a memory and started my brain to react. My lungs expand but I can't breathe. An elephant plops on my chest.

Don't breathe.

Don't look.

Don't see.

Don't hear.

This must be what it is like. No breath, no life, emptiness, nothing.

Like lilac.

———————

Sybil had to be wrong about what would happen in the operating room. I knew that Mr. Allen had to go to the operating room. But if Sybil were right, might he have a cardiac arrest and die? Would I hear that there was a Code in the CAT scan suite? Would I hear, Code Blue, CAT scan suite? Code Blue, CAT scan suite, Code Blue, CAT scan suite.

The scent of lilac. I sniffed and smelled and sniffed again. Death to me was lilac. I quietly sniffed to smell if it was all around me. This reaction to the scent was unusual. Lilac was used at funerals as it was a symbol of love. But the association between the two was etched in my brain.

No.

Nothing.

No lilac.

No smell.

Just nothing.

CHAPTER 4

I SEE UNUSUAL THINGS

M y eyes shot open and I stared into the entry way of the bedroom door. It was the middle of the afternoon and I had fallen asleep on Donald's bed. I was awake and I was trying to move. I needed to get up. But, I could not move. My feet would not budge. My hands were paralyzed. I could not lift my head off the bed. My entire body was weighed down. The man in the doorway stared at me. He was smiling. At least it looked like a smile.

His complexion was the palest alabaster white. His hair was jet black, wavy, and touched the tip of his shoulders. He could have easily put his hair into a ponytail, but he wore it straight out. He was balding in the middle, but he did not sweep strands of hair over the spot to cover it up. He held a hat in his hand. His forehead was high, broad, and his nose was straight, full, and thick. The tip of his nostrils flared. Depending on the angle from which you viewed him, the flare could be a smile or a snarl. He was conscious of that potential misinterpretation. Therefore, he held his head so that it was a smile.

His eyes were steely grey. They were not human eyes and belonged to a wolf. They were deep, focused, and intense. Or were the eyes blue? I could not really tell. Or maybe they were brown or green? I did not recognize the color, but I must have seen that color before. I did not want to take a second look. He was neatly dressed in a white shirt, black tie, and black trousers. His clothes had no wrinkles. He smiled and showed perfectly shaped teeth with no gaps between them. He stood at the door staring at me for what seemed like more than an eternity. The flare of the nose did not change. This was the nose's natural shape and not a sign of disdain or anger.

I tried to smile in return but found that I could not. I would not. It appeared that no muscle in my body could move. Was I just paralyzed by fear from the grey-blue-brown-what-ever-color eyes that stared? I must still be asleep. But, wait, no, my eyes were open and I was looking directly at the man in the doorway. I was seeing clearly and my eyes were open. When he saw that I would not return the smile he tried to stop smiling too. But the angle of the head and the flare of the nose left him with a perpetual smile.

I closed my eyes and commanded my body, "Move! Move!"

By the time I opened my eyes again the man in the door was gone. I willed my body to move. "Move. Move," I said. "Move arms. Move legs. Move," I commanded.

"Get up. Move."

I must have been dreaming but now I was awake. But nothing changed. No part of my body would work. I took a deep breath and closed my eyes again. I opened my eyes and oops, now my hands moved. And my legs moved. I sat bolt upright with my heart racing and beating fast against my chest. I was not sweating but I felt a fire burning with the continuous drum beat pounding of my heart. I jumped off the bed and ran outside with my heart now pushed to beat and pound much faster from running.

Donald was stooped over a circle drawn in the dirt. He quickly knocked a small red marble against the yellow multicolored one and it landed nicely in the center of the circle. He was still playing marbles against himself. I guess he had continued playing alone after I must have gone inside for something, and fallen asleep on his bed.

"Hey, where did that man go?" I asked Donald.

"What man?" Donald asked.

"You know, the man with the white shirt. He had a black tie on. The one who was in the house."

Donald snapped some more marbles into the ring. His pants pockets were now bulging with his winnings as he was beating the invisible competitor.

"There is no man. My mother is in her room and I am out here," Donald said.

"There is no man here. There is no one else here," he repeated.

"Oh. But what about the man who had on the white shirt and black tie? His eyes were grey or blue. He had a big forehead and his nose was straight but thick."

"What are you talking about?"

"I saw him just now."

"No you did not. Uncle Jim has been dead since I don't even know when. It must have been last year or the year before, oh, I don't know when. Where did you see him?" Donald asked, looking at me with a strange look as he was asking again.

"In the house, as I told you."

"You are out of your mind!" Donald said, with more emphasis than was really necessary based on what I had just told him.

"You cannot see Uncle Jim, he is dead," Donald snorted and said and rolled his eyes up into his head.

"Oh," I said, completely deflated and confused and not knowing what else to say or do right then.

I blankly stared at him and did not say anything more. I looked at the ground and then glanced into the sky. Sam, my brother, had told my mother that he had seen Grandma Bea and that she had spoken to him. My mother had said that Sam was making that up.

"You cannot see Grandma Bea. She's dead," my mother said. "Remember, Sam, we went to the funeral. She is in heaven, she is not here anymore, and is gone forever." My mother then turned again to Sam, saying, "Don't ever tell anyone if you see dead people or that they spoke to you. People will think that you've lost it. Don't say that again. You hear?"

"You hear me? People will think that you are not in your right mind. Do you understand that, what I just said?" she asked.

Sam nodded in silence. So, if he ever saw a dead person again or if they spoke to him he would not tell anyone. Sam decided he would not ever tell anyone then, not even Mom. Mom must have meant that message for me too, I thought. "A lesson that you did not learn," I said to myself.

"Oh," I said loudly.

"No, you cannot see dead people. No one can," Donald said.

"Oh. Oh?"

Praying Women

I don't know why my mind had catapulted me all the way back to my childhood. I was not under any more stress than usual. I was not being bullied, harassed or feeling as if I was being subjected to danger or bodily harm. There was no scent of lilac that reminded me of death. I was not having an asthma attack. I was able to breathe well. But I must have been holding my breath. But, I was not breathing deeply and fully.

"C-two, three, four, keep the diaphragm alive," I said to myself. Breathe, breathe, breathe, breathe. That was the mnemonic that we used in medical school to remember that the cervical nerves, the second, third, and fourth nerves, coming from the neck in the cervical spine, helped you to breathe. The nerves made the diaphragms move. The diaphragm was the muscle that moved up and down to expand the lungs so that you could breathe. If the nerves were not working you would not breathe.

"C-2, 3, 4, breathe, breathe, breathe!" I encouraged myself.

Sam pitched forward and almost fell trying to cross the doorway. Instantly, I remembered the task that was at hand. I was trying to get Sam into the house in his drunken state, but he had tripped on the one step that he had to step on to get into the house from the garage. I must have been holding my breath to avoid inhaling the aroma, grassy smell and accumulated sweat that was coming from Sam's body. I was trying not to get intoxicated myself from that whiff of alcohol. Sam had drunk too much alcohol all day.

It must have been a long time since Sam had a drink. That's as far as I knew anyway. I did not keep any alcohol in the house at all. There was no reason to add any other temptation to an already toxic mix. Besides, Sam was taking several medications. It would not be a good idea to mix alcohol with his pills. If we had any events or holiday celebrations at home, I brought only sufficient alcohol to do a toast, or whatever was needed. After that, I would give what remained to the guests or simply dumped the rest down the drain.

The short ride home had not sobered Sam up enough for him to be fully awake. He still needed help to go up the steps. I propped him up on the right side to make him be somewhat upright. He was still walking with a bent gait. I helped him up and got him to the foot of the stairs. I egged him on to slowly step up each step. By the time we had made it up the fifteen steps and turned on the second floor landing I was out of breath. God, I have got to get to the gym and get physically active. Sitting and remaining inactive all day was not good. My excuse was all those twelve hour shifts in the emergency room. I thought because I spent so much time running back and forth in the hallways that was sufficient. It was not. Besides, with all that running that I did to respond to Code Blues and the trauma room? You've got to be kidding me? After that and I was still not in shape? I felt that I had already done a million miles in one day. If I did not do a million miles daily, it certainly had to be at least a million steps. That probably was an exaggeration but it seemed like a million. I told myself to remember to get a pedometer to wear on my belt daily. Keeping physically active was good. It certainly did not necessarily mean that I had to go work out in a gym three times a week. From now on, walking more would be just what I needed to keep in better shape.

I finally got Sam into his bedroom and he sat on his bed.

"Look, there is no way I can get you into the shower tonight."

"Let me take off your clothes, Sam. We can do the rest in the morning. By that time you should be sober. Then we can figure out what to do."

I had to get him back to the assisted living center. He had to go back, at least for now. There was no way that I could work my shifts in the emergency room and come home to take care of him. That plan was not working. I needed to figure out the next best steps. In no time Sam was asleep on the bed. I left him there sleeping and walked to my room. I had to think about what to do next.

I thought back to the time when I first knew that something was not quite right with Sam. I was only about eight years old. I had just come home from school in the afternoon. I was heading to the kitchen to get some juice and a snack. I then heard voices whispering and praying. I went to look from where the voices were coming. I peeked into the living room as the hushed voices were coming from there. Sam sat in the middle of a circle with about six women surrounding him. The women were praying and alternately touching him on his head. They were reading scriptures and singing. They asked God to heal and touch Sam and to make him whole. Some of them prayed out loudly. Others were quiet with their pleas. But their zeal was evident. I felt then that this was a serious problem. Maybe it required an intervention from an outside power. We always talked about healing the mind, body, and spirit. Maybe this was a spiritual problem.

Sam had been home because he had not gone to school for the week. I had overheard our mother say that she had to find a new school for him. This was yet another one. It was probably the fifth school in less than two years. Something must have happened at school. I had seen enough and I had heard enough. I could not make out besides the healing what else the women were asking for. I walked away to the kitchen to get something, but by the time I got there I had forgotten whatever it was I wanted there. Yes, something had not been quite right all along.

My reverie was interrupted by the sudden need to get the alcohol smell off me. I went to the shower in my bathroom and had to soap up twice to wash away the alcohol and rancid smell from me. I think subconsciously I was hoping to wash away the memories of the past and all the events of trying to find him after Charlie had called me to find Sam. I had to figure out what to do next. But what was that?

Egg Sandwich

I was a fairly good cook as I had gotten lots of practice. They say that after you have done something for at least ten thousand hours you are considered an expert. I must have been an expert by the age of ten. I had gotten lots of practice by preparing and cooking meals for myself. But, I hated cooking, and I hated being in the kitchen.

Since Sam lived with me I did not let him cook anything at all. First, his attention was poor. I feared that he would put a pot on the stove and just leave it there to burn. Second, the muscles in his right hand were contracted and weak. He could barely lift and move the pots and pans. Moreover, I did not want him near fire or sharp objects. I did not keep any sharp knives visible in the kitchen. When someone came to our house and wanted to use the kitchen, I had to be there to give them everything. I locked away anything sharp. It was just easier if everyone else stayed out of the kitchen. Maybe I was being paranoid over it, but they say prevention is better than cure. I would rather practice that first, and I wanted to keep it that way.

As far as meals were concerned I planned ahead. I tried to make meal preparation less of a chore and more of a routine. I prepared everything for the week on Saturdays or Sundays. I would cook three different items— chicken, beef, and seafood. Once these items were prepared, I froze the rest to be thawed and warmed up during the week. Variety was not on the menu. In the midst of potential chaos simplicity is welcomed. I was not one to complain about consistency. I was happy to eat the same thing over and over and never get bored by it. My friends laughed at how I could eat the same bland thing twice. Practice makes perfect. Perfect peace was even more perfect. Not to rock the boat was fine by me.

I loved to eat an egg sandwich. It was the easiest thing to prepare and in a minute you could be out of the kitchen. I also loved Fridays. On Fridays we did not cook a full meal and we made eggs for dinner. Fried eggs, scrambled eggs, eggs sunny side up or down or soft or hard boiled eggs. It was your choice. I liked my eggs fully cooked and made into an egg sandwich. When our parents' friends came to visit, my parents would say, "Gary, make them an egg sandwich."

With the exception for making the egg sandwich, I stayed as far away from the kitchen as possible. It got too hot in there and I hated the smell of food being prepared. After the meal was prepared I would be glad to eat it. However, the scent of lilac and the scent of food in preparation were my Achilles' heel. Therefore, as far as Fridays go, this was a typical Friday. But, on this particular Friday, around six o'clock in the evening, our mother peaked into our bedrooms.

"You guys are on your own. I need to take Sam to the hospital," Mom said. "Sam is having an asthma attack."

I did not think too much about any of it. It was Friday and I was used to fending for myself. It was Friday and the kitchen would be hot as the day was very warm. I was satisfied with my egg sandwich. What else was new? Sam was always getting asthma attacks, and Esther always took him to the hospital to get it treated.

Sam was now about seventeen years old. School had always been a problem for him. By the time he was that age he had been in and out of several schools. I don't think he lasted for more than a year at any of the schools. He would constantly get into fights and they said he was a troublemaker. He would not listen to any of the teachers. He never did any homework, from what I saw. He spoke in riddles and I could not follow the reasoning. At other times you saw him staring into space for no reason that was obvious to anyone. He would stand in one place and in one position for a long period of time. Sometimes, he would suddenly begin to speak loudly. Who was he talking to? I knew that he was not talking to me, and there was no one else there. Who was he having the conversation with?

I was not surprised when Esther came back with Marilyn, her sister. Marilyn had gone to the hospital with Esther and they were both angry. Sam tricked them as he was not having an asthma attack. Or if he had, by the time he got there, and saw that woman, the asthma attack left him. He saw that woman and loudly laughed out.

The woman had been standing in the middle of the emergency room. She was thin, exquisitely contoured and looked like a ballerina. Her neck was long and she held her head high. Her limbs were thin like spokes of a bicycle wheel. A complex pattern of sinuous veins crisscrossed her forearms. Her scapula and shoulder blades protruded, and every major and minor muscle in her upper back was evident. Her finger nails were filled with grime and dirt. They had no nail polish on them. She stood there in the middle of the room without moving for what seemed like an eternity. She stood there quietly, like horses would, then unexpectedly she would lift one foot up then the other down. They listened to hear the stomping of hooves. None came. When she walked though, she still moved in a jerky manner, but it was still graceful.

From her physical appearance you expected her movements to be more fluid and effortless. Her shoulders and hips were narrow, and her clavicles were prominent forming a perfect cleft on each side. Every fashion model would have envied her bone structure. Her back was straight, and she stood upright with good posture, except she rolled her shoulders downwards. The weight of the world must have been on them. Her knees were narrow and her calf muscles were well developed. Her feet were small and narrow. She wore sandals that had some of the straps missing. Her big toes had bunions and the other toes had callouses. The toenails were chipped and uneven. A podiatrist would have squealed with delight to be able to bring those feet back to their former beauty. She was definitely too thin. She appeared as if she missed the next glass of water, or another meal, she would collapse unconscious on the floor, exhausted from dehydration.

She must have been homeless. Her clothes were tattered. Her blouse hung loosely on her body. She wore pants that were held to her waist with cords that were twisted into an intricate design. Her hair was in its natural state but the tresses were matted and mangled together. Some of the tresses spiked upwards creating the effect of a tiara. Her skin was the complexion of the deepest mahogany. It would have been unblemished except for the acne scattered on her forehead and cheeks. She wore heavy makeup and her lips were firebox red from over-applied lipstick. Once she had been absolutely beautiful. You knew now that her mind was completely gone. But you also knew that at one point in time she was able to stop people in their tracks to stare when she walked into a room. She still had that same effect on them.

When Sam laughed out loud and pointed at her she turned to face the sound. She twirled and twirled as a dancer would to entertain her audience. Her eyes were oval shaped and she looked way off into the distance. She did not appear to be here in this place. Her eyes though were soft and kind. Just as suddenly as she had twirled, she stopped as a windup ballerina on a jewel box would have. She moved away from the other patients sitting in the waiting room to stand alone in a corner. She continued to murmur to herself and to have a conversation with an invisible stranger.

When Sam laughed his asthma attack must have gone away. Esther and Marilyn were furious that they had taken him there for no reason. If Sam could have laughed out that loudly obviously, he was not that sick. They then said that the asthma attack was simply a ruse to avoid chores. He had wasted their time in the emergency room again. They were convinced that his asthma attack was an emotional response to something else, and not a real problem.

But when Sam laughed at the dancing woman it may have been that he felt a connection with her. It may have been recognition of a kinship that he did not know existed. In ten years or less he too would have been homeless, hungry, emaciated, and physically unrecognizable. His mind would have unraveled. His thoughts would become jumbled, his speech incoherent, and his judgment impaired. He too would be hearing voices and seeing things that did not exist. His movements would also become jerky and his gait stiff. He would stare outward with a blank and flat expression and his eyes would not engage you. He would not make any eye contact. You would speak to him and you would not be sure that he heard you or understood what was being said.

Esther and Marilyn knew that something was wrong with Sam. Was it a problem with the body or the mind? On that occasion they did not think Sam had a problem with the body. They did not believe that his asthma attack was real. The pieces did not fit.

After hearing about that incident in the emergency room it came as no surprise when a couple of days later I saw Sam standing in the bathroom. Usually, he took too much time in the bathroom anyway. I found it unusual that when he went into the bathroom to only have a bowel movement that he had to take off all of his clothes. No one that we knew got completely naked just to use the toilet. But that was Sam. This time though he was not naked. He stood fixed looking into the bathroom mirror and he held scissors in his right hand. Clumps of his black hair lay at his feet. There were single and multiple strands of his curly black hair intertwined with the rug. The hair style he was creating was still a work in progress. Sam had unevenly chopped off different parts of his hair while making his haircut. The style was jagged and haphazard.

He was staring into the mirror in front of him; therefore, he should have been able to see what he was doing. But sometimes looking into a parallel universe may make you disoriented. All the hair on the left side was chopped off in a sharp, triangulated fashion.

Snip, snip, snip.

Chop, chop, chop.

Sam chopped at the remaining hair some more. Some more strands of hair fell to the rug and other strands splattered on the tiled floor. I looked into the bathroom mirror to see who in the parallel universe held his attention. Was there someone on the other side? If there was, I could not make him out. Yet, Sam stared into the mirror, chopping and snipping, snipping and chopping. The person on the other side must have commanded him to do it. He must have told Sam to chop and snip his hair in that way. I slowly backed away from the bathroom door and immediately started to yell out.

"Mom, Mom. Come see, come see. Sam is cutting off all of his hair. Sam is cutting his hair off. Come see what he did," I begged.

Mom ran towards me and into the bathroom to see Sam's new haircut. She had to see. She stepped quickly into the bathroom and took one look at Sam. Without flinching, she grabbed the scissors out of his hands, and Sam toddled backwards trying to prevent the steal.

"Stop it, stop it!" she screamed.

"Stop it and go to your room, now!"

"Gary. You too. Go to your room now!"

What did I do? All I did was to raise the alarm? What would she have done if I had not called her to action? By the time Sam was done all the hair would have been gone? Why did I now have to go my room? Our mother glared at Sam not understanding what had just happened.

"Why did he just cut his hair off? What nonsense is this? What is his problem? What's the matter with him?" she asked.

"I must take him to the hospital, again," she said under her breath muttering to herself.

"This is much too much to bear."

Hair Day

On Saturdays, I wish I would be like Sam and not be able to sit still for long periods of time. At nights now, he would constantly move and pace when everyone was sleeping, or trying to sleep. He would pace constantly back and forth in our bedroom and would talk to himself. Nowadays, all his arms and legs and limbs had to be in constant motion. He would mutter to himself then would stop suddenly in the middle of the room. He would stop talking and walking, and he would be listening to someone. They could not hear or did not understand. He would then say in a loud voice, "No, I am not going to do that." Apparently, they had not heard him the first time, and therefore, he repeated it even louder. "No, I said, I am not going to do that!" What were they commanding him to do?

I, on the other hand, could stay still, but this was not to my advantage. On Saturdays, Fatima, our cousin, a hairstylist, and who lived with us, would style wigs for her friends. She did not have a mannequin or a plastic head to style the wigs on, so, I was it. I was the living styling head. Everyone else would be off having fun but I was at work. I sat quietly and Fatima would twist and turn the chair around, back and forth, left then right, as I sat there with the wig on my head. My head burned, my thoughts fried, my mind scrambled. I wanted to scratch to get free and fling the thing off my head.

"No, no." Fatima said. "No."

I closed my eyes and longed to reach up to yank that weight off. I wanted to be free.

"Don't even try it. Don't even try it. You can't move and you can't touch the hair. Look, you just destroyed the style!" Fatima yelled.

"Don't move! Don't you dare move!" Fatima said. "Otherwise, I have to start from scratch," she said.

"Okay. Okay. So, move and spin the chair then," I said to myself.

I thought about school and what I learned there. I closed my eyes and dreamed about the places I learned about in geography. I dreamed about the sky and committed the planets to memory. I dreamed not to be in this place. But this experience also taught me the power of being still. I slowed my own activity down. I don't think Sam could as easily control what he felt and what he did. Was it a problem of the mind or body? Was there a problem in his brain connections so that the brain could not self-correct and control itself?

Being still taught me that in being quiet you can silently dream and think about all the things in your life. It helped me to love the loudness of thought in the stillness of peace.

TIP BOX 1

1. Health: Your First Priority is your health. See your doctor and follow the recommended prevention guidelines

2. Priority: everything cannot be a priority. Your check-list should be at most, only three items. Nothing comes on to the check-list unless something is moved off

3. Quiet time: take time to remain still and reflect on where you have been, where you want to go, and create an action plan on how to get there

PART II

CHARTING THE COURSE

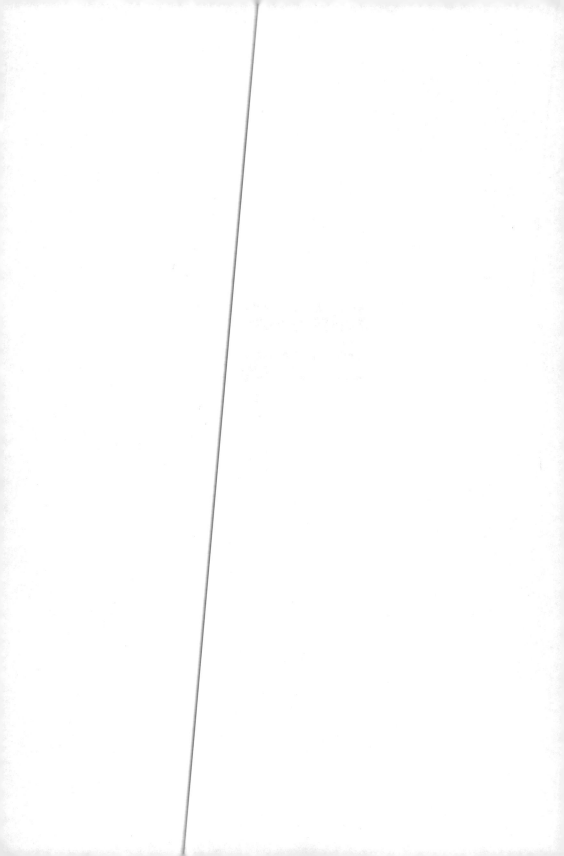

Bull's eye

Quiver, quake
Pulled and strained
You brought me deep
To take me wide
The trajectory to see
Bent to the point of break
You made the arc
My life would take
Palpate, shake
Tremble and take
Yield to your will
Sharpened by your skill
A point of rest before the flight
To hit the mark
The bull's eye test.

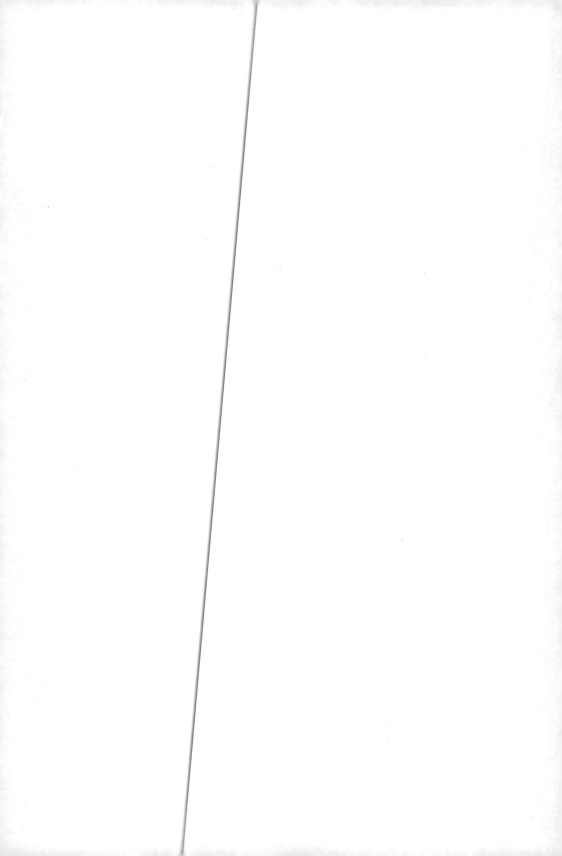

CHAPTER 5

FISH TAIL CAR

D orian was not at school for the entire spring term and no one knew what happened to him. Therefore, Sam had gotten a break from the bullying as Dorian was the ringleader. If Dorian were not there the other students tended to be more tolerant of Sam and his unusual behaviors.

"Where is Dorian?" everyone had asked. All the students had secretly hoped that he had changed schools. It would have been better still if he had gone to another planet. Sam at least hoped so anyway even if no one else had.

Sam was happy that Dorian was not there and he hoped Dorian would end up any place else in the universe except back in the school. At least for now Sam could use his pocket change to buy what he wanted at lunch. He was happy to have a choice of buying and eating something other than the unrecognizable school lunch, and much more than that, Sam was grateful for not having more sand thrown in his eyes. The break from that was good, but that period of calm did not last too long.

In September, Dorian came back to school to rule the school yard. But he came in on crutches. Sam said that Dorian told them that he had been hit by a car. He had been crossing the street at Retirement Crescent and apparently, he had not looked left or right. As he stepped off the curb, the blue fish-tailed car came barreling towards him. He said he flew up into the air and crashed down into the middle of the street. Luckily no other cars were coming for that would have been the end of him. He said that he lay in the street not being able to move. His lower body was all broken up. He had survived the hit but had broken his pelvis and the bones in his legs.

"Yes. I am lucky to be alive," Dorian said.

After Sam had told me that story I looked out for cars. I constantly looked out for the blue car with fish tail. I did not want to become the next victim with a broken leg. I became so obsessed that I would look right then left, then right then left, then right again, before stepping off any curb. I was becoming paralyzed by my own fear that I was forgetting to live my life.

Therefore, as I thought about that childhood memory, I tried to remain calm as I watched the man ignore our orders for the tenth time. We had asked him to remain still on the stretcher. There was an expected level of common courtesy and professionalism that is ingrained when you work with the public. Customer service was important and we all got evaluated on that in emergency room work. But sometimes, there is just that one person who continually pushes the envelope. He provokes you and skates out onto thin ice. The professional expectation is that you ignore all of that. You are there to practice medicine and to save his life. Despite the irritation that you feel you have to still be nice. But, how long should you watch someone potentially do harm to themselves and not do anything? Should you remain calm, cool, collected? Do you stand by and smile sweetly and continue being nice? How do you know when too much is really too much? Do you draw a firm line in the sand at the start and not allow anyone to even come close to it or even cross it?

Such was the dilemma with the young man that was just brought into the emergency room after a car crash. My patience was now super thin. I felt myself grinding my teeth. I looked around the room and everyone's facial expression was fixed in concrete. We had asked in one way or another for him to wait a moment. "Please be still so that we can get our jobs done." But, I had had enough by the eleventh time that someone had asked him to remain still so that we could do our work.

"Enough already!" I said.

"*Basta ya!*" I added.

"*Arretez-vous la!*" I said to communicate with him in any language possible. Maybe he did not understand English.

"Lie down now," I said.

"I said, NOW!"

A CORE trauma had been called for the car crash. I was the emergency room physician who had come to the trauma room, and the trauma surgeons were also on their way. In a minute or two the surgical residents were also all streaming into the trauma bay.

The young man, who the ambulance crew had brought in, was the driver in the car crash. The crew had placed a plastic cervical collar to secure his neck. That was meant to protect his cervical spine, the seven bones in his neck, from an injury. The ambulance crew was trying to tell us about the crash. If they told us more about what the crash scene looked like, we could think about the types of injuries that he may have. The nurses and surgical residents were busy trying to cut off his clothes so that we could fully examine him. We needed to see if he had any injuries. One of the nurses on his right side was asking him to stay still. She was trying to put an IV in so that she could get blood-work. She may also need to give him give medications and hang saline. But, he kept thrashing around on the bed and sitting up on the stretcher. Nothing and no one could get him to stop moving. Ryan, another nurse at the bedside, had just gotten an IV on the left side. He had barely secured it with tape, gauze, and a transparent cover when the guy sat up again. The cervical collar was becoming loose, dangling from his neck.

"It was not my fault, it was not my fault," he screamed.

"Get down, stay down, lie down now," I insisted. "Ryan, please secure the collar and hold his neck."

Rick, the ambulance attendant, showed me the picture of the car. The front end was completely smashed like an accordion and it appeared as if the engine ended up in the driver's seat.

"Wow," I said to no one in particular.

"You have to lie down so that we can examine you and see if you have any injuries."

"Take this mess off my neck," he said.

"Look, you have to lie down now."

"Get this mess off my neck," he screamed.

"That mess is on your neck to protect it. It will save your life. Don't even touch that mess," I said. I knew that all that talking was a waste of time. I simply knew he was not going to cooperate.

"Mother, get this off me?"

"Hey, hey, hey, don't talk to us like that," I said. He went on with a string of expletives.

"Okay. Okay. Do you have any allergies?" I asked.

"Do you take any medications?"

"Were you drinking or doing any drugs?"

"Marijuana, cocaine, heroin, PCP, Ecstasy? Anything? Anything at all?"

"Are you dusted? Are you on Spice?" I asked.

"Dusted" was the slang for being under the influence of "angel dust," PCP, which is phencyclidine. The use of synthetic marijuana or cannabis was also on the increase. This synthetic herbal and chemical product was said to mimic the effects of marijuana. It was psychoactive, meaning that it had effects on the brain when it was used. It was usually used by smoking. It was also commonly known as K2 and Spice. Synthetic cannabis was often referred to as the "spice product." The terms K2 and Spice were now being used in general to refer to this type of manufactured, synthetic, marijuana.

There was enough information to link marijuana use with acute psychosis. A psychosis means a mental breakdown where users were not able to distinguish reality. The user could start to have hallucinations of hearing or seeing things that were not there, not present at all. There was also research being done on the safety of synthetic cannabis. The initial studies were trying to focus on whether synthetic marijuana could result in psychosis. The studies did seem to suggest that synthetic cannabis can precipitate psychosis, and in some cases the psychosis lasts a very long time. Just as with marijuana, it appeared that the synthetic form of the drug could make a person who previously had a stable psychotic disorder much worse. It was also possible that, like marijuana, the factory made form could trigger a chronic, long-term, psychotic disorder. This was especially true in vulnerable persons, in those at highest risk, such as those with a family history of mental illness. There was a link between marijuana use and the onset or provoking schizophrenia.

The patient was out of control. He must have been "dusted" or "spiced" up. If not that then he must have been "liquored up." In either case, the next plan was B. We had no time for him to hurt himself and maybe even hurt us.

"You need to lie down now and be still. Otherwise, it's good night, have a nice sleep, and we will see you in the morning," I said. I signaled to Ryan to get the tray ready.

"Enough already! *Basta ya! Arretez-vous la!*" I looked over to Dr. Luke Jones. "Yikes! This one takes the cake! Enough already!" I repeated.

"No. No. No. Enough. He needs RSI now!"

Luke Jones was a newly minted surgical doctor. He was older than most doctors when they had finished all their training, and was able to work without supervision. He had finished high school on time and had always wanted to be a doctor. He had gotten into college to pursue a pre-medical course of training. But, somewhere along the way life distracted him, as it tends to do. He spent the summer between high school and college working. When it was time for him to go off to college that fall, he did not go and he kept on working. Eventually he became an ED tech, working in the emergency room helping the nurses with chores, doing EKGs and whatever else the nurses asked him to do. He worked as a tech and found time to go to nursing school at night and on his days off from work.

Luke always seemed to be involved in some type of educational activity, and worked for two years as a nurse. That gave him some flexibility to work different shifts and study at the same time. He had taken the medical college admissions tests, MCATs, had performed well, and was accepted into medical school. It was good to see him come back to the hospital as a surgical resident and he had just completed his five years of surgical residency training. He was now the surgeon coming to the trauma call. He was an excellent physician with superb technical skills. But in addition, he had an excellent bed-side manner and had the patience of Job. I think because his path to becoming a surgeon was not typical, it made him a patient person. His road to this point was filled with twists and turns, and he learned the power of perseverance. The tapestry of his life must have been quite colorful and changing, but he held onto his dream to be a surgeon.

"Enough already!" I said again.

"We need to intubate him so that we can do our work," I said. Luke nodded his agreement.

"RSI, now. Enough already!" I repeated. I performed the rapid sequence intubation, also called RSI. The first medication was an amnestic and sedative so that the patient would not remember anything. In seconds he would be asleep. We had no choice up to this point. There was no other way for us to examine him and to see if he had any injuries from the crash.

I then gave the muscle relaxant, which would stop his breathing, and I then put the breathing tube into his trachea. This was a small plastic tube that went in the mouth and into the airway. After that was done we could control his breathing. Finally, the trauma team could examine him and look at his chest, back, arms, and legs to see if anything was wrong.

He was now "tubed" and the respiratory technician attached the tube to the ventilator, the machine that would control his breathing. Finally, we could get the CAT scans of his body. At that point we had to scan him from hem to stern. We would scan the head, neck, chest, abdomen, and pelvis to see if there were any injuries. Now that he was unconscious we could get our job done. Ryan placed a second IV in his right arm while the surgical residents continued to look him over. They did ultrasounds of the internal organs before going to the CAT scan machine looking for internal bleeding or other problems. We looked for any shadows or layering of fluid to be sure that there was no free blood, air, or shattered organs. We found nothing abnormal on the ultrasound but the ultrasound was only the start. We had to continue to search to be sure that there was not something seriously wrong. I called the CAT technician to tell her that we were bringing over a "tubed" trauma patient.

"Hey, Cheryl. What's up? We got one for you. We need him pan-scanned, from head to toe," I said.

The alcohol level came back and it was three times above the legal level for what is considered driving under the influence. He had been drinking and driving drunk.

Rick, the ambulance crew attendant, chimed in.

"I think he was texting and not paying attention too," Rick said.

"I saw his open phone on the car seat when we extracted him from the car. And it looked like he was texting as I could see that he had a long thread of conversation. It looks like he had not responded to one text that had just come in. And to add insult to injury, he had alcohol on board too?" Rick asked.

"I don't even think he was wearing a seatbelt," Rick added.

There were many injuries that the guy could have. He might have been drinking and texting, and that would have made him completely distracted. I guessed that he was not wearing a seatbelt and that he was driving fast. If he had hit his chest on the steering wheel, he could have broken his breast bone, clavicle or ribs. One of the worse injuries could be if he had ripped his aorta, the large blood vessel coming off his heart that supplies blood to the rest of the body. The aorta obviously was not totally ruptured because he would have been dead on the scene or his blood pressure would have been low. Nevertheless, he was thrashing about, sitting up on the stretcher and not listening to us. This made it difficult for the team to figure out what was wrong. Intubating him and putting him to sleep was the right decision.

Driving your car while distracted is driving while doing another activity and that takes your attention away from driving. That simple act can increase the chance of having a motor vehicle crash. First, there were the two major distractions: cell phone use and texting. As I drive now, I see too many people on their cell phones or texting. What is so important that it cannot wait until you get to your destination? Is it such an emergency? Why not pull off to the side of the road and take the call? I didn't want to have to see them on a stretcher all broken up.

The distractions are a triple threat to you and others. It is a visual, manual, and cognitive threat. It is visual in the sense that you are taking your eyes off the road and the cars and objects ahead of you. It is manual because you are taking your hands off the wheel. And finally it was cognitive because you are taking your mind off what you are doing.

Too many drivers use the cell phone, text, and eat when driving. Using in-vehicle technologies, such as navigation systems, can also be sources of distraction. Any of these distractions can endanger the driver and others. But texting while driving is especially dangerous because it combines all three types of distraction. This is really a huge problem.

Distracted driving was a triple threat. This was not the performing arts where a triple threat is a good thing. If you can act, sing, and dance all equally well, well good for you. But the triple threat of distracted driving was likely to have a bad outcome.

I was glad that I put the breathing tube in the patient. First, I had no choice. I needed to do my job and save his life. Here was another trauma code in the emergency room that was unnecessary. I had to find the code for sanity. This man needed a good night's sleep. I hoped that when he awoke the next day that he would be refreshed and ready to start anew. Would he think about his actions and their effect on himself and on others? Would he do that for himself, for his family, and for others?

CHAPTER 6

DYLAN'S HOOP DREAM

I was walking with Dylan from the dorm to go to dinner in the dining hall. I was lost in my own reverie about unusual events, and listening to Dylan talk about basketball. I admit I was only half-listening. I was thinking about Sam and how he said that there were extraterrestrials and invisible people being all over the place. In a way, I thought that since I was used to the unusual, that should help me to adjust to college, not be afraid of meeting new people, and trying new endeavors.

Sam said that he felt the ETs. He entertained and spoke with them. Somehow, they did not want to be ignored. I never personally had that experience, and was grateful, as Sam said the ETs were a crafty bunch. They morphed into different people and different forms. Moreover, they were very selective with the company that they kept as they only revealed themselves to a few people.

The ETs used aliases. Sam called them a number of things—UFO, the Martians, the Green People, or John Canoe. But, by whatever name they went by, only Sam could see or hear them. They appeared several times to Sam and I could tell when there was a visit. I knew something was up when the voices started as Sam's behavior would change. He became very quiet or very talkative. Sam would get a wild look in his eyes, and his eyes would open up wide, like giant-sized pods where you could see all the white of his eyes. His pupils would dilate fully as one's eyes do when trying to see in the dark, or when the eyes behold something of beauty or interest. His face would contort, and the facial muscles would tighten, and gain definition. He would tilt his head to one side as if he were listening to someone speaking to him. It was almost as in a conspiracy, as he leaned in closer to hear what they were saying.

If necessary, to listen intently, he tilted his head more. And, if it seemed that they were speaking in too much of a hushed tone, he leaned in, and moved in closer. At such times, it must have been difficult for Sam to hear them as they were speaking so lowly. I never heard the voices speak and I never saw the owners of the voice. No one else around seemed to hear them either. At times you could see Sam shaking his head, as if to say that he did not agree with the invisibles, or maybe that he just wanted them to shut up and go away.

Therefore, I thought I would be prepared for anything. I was wrong. Dylan and I were just about to walk into the dining hall to get dinner when seven or eight girls stopped us on the cobbled path leading to the dining hall. The girls were giggling amongst themselves. We stopped as they blocked our way into the cafeteria. Without them moving, which they had no intention of doing, we were compelled to take part in whatever they had in mind. They kept on giggling and laughing in their conspiracy.

"Oh, we want to rate you and give you a score," they said in unison. "Do you all mind?" They squealed in delight to seal the deal.

I shrugged, "Who cares?"

Dylan said, "Yes, sure." He answered too quickly even before he knew exactly what they were up to. I went along with it, "Who cares? You can give me a number if you want," I thought.

Dylan smiled, squared out his shoulders, and puffed up his chest. He straightened up and posed. Well, all that posturing was totally unnecessary as he played basketball and was athletic. His hair was neatly cropped to his too perfectly shaped head. Everyone said he was good looking and he knew it. So all that posing and flexing was totally not necessary and not really called for in this or any situation. I stood straight up too. I was five feet eight but too skinny, too lanky, and my teenager's acne was splotched all over my face. I did not play basketball but played tennis. Well, I had before coming to college. I played tennis in high school but did not play now, the second semester in college. I had gotten too busy with studying, reading, and with classes to bother with tennis now. No one would ever call me an athlete.

Anyway, Esther, my mother, had warned, "You can't do both, play sports, and study, so which is it?"

"I don't see any doctor ever playing tennis. Ever. They don't play football or basketball either," Esther said. "Golf maybe," she said. "But for now, you can't do both."

My teachers thought I should be a doctor. They pushed me to take chemistry, physics, and calculus. I barely explored classes in English or literature, but even there the teachers recommended sticking to the sciences. Sometimes, you don't know where the path is taking you, but becoming a doctor helped me to understand the complex medical issues that I would eventually face.

But that was high school and this is college. And everybody here said and knew that high school didn't count for anything, not right here, and not now. This was a new place with new friends and new challenges. You had to claim a new case in college and start from scratch. Being able to adapt to change is essential. Change is constant in life, and when it came it required resiliency. Sometimes it meant that you had to bend to the point of break. To reduce the stresses with change you could either adapt or avoid. Being on this campus, there was no way to avoid it, and I quickly learned to adapt.

Dylan was still posing. What was he so concerned about? He knew that they will give him a fifteen or twenty, out of the maximum possible ten. They conspired some more and giggled again as they tried to figure out what score their compatriots would give each of us. I tried to stand a little bit straighter and stronger still. Each girl put Dylan's scores up.

Dylan had worked hard too as he had been an athlete all his life. He loved sports, and loved to entertain, and we hooped and hollered when our school was winning in any game and at any sport. And we, as spectators, were jumping with joy and laughing and loved to watch them smash the other teams and win by even a measly one point. Winning was better than losing. The higher the score, the better it was. But now he was in college and studying like everyone else.

His years of playing sports taught him many things. He followed a fitness routine to become physically ready. The coaches talked a lot about practicing and having discipline. Dylan usually played a team sport and each player was given a role to play. He knew what it was like to be on a team. The members of the team had to play together to increase the chance of winning. The coaches always showed them the game plan and how to follow it. On game day the players followed the game plan, and when things went wrong it was either because the game plan was wrong or someone did not follow the game plan. It was either a wrong strategy or wrong execution or both. Dylan transferred what he learned on the playing fields into the classrooms. Therefore, he was no academic slouch.

The girls put my scores up.

I accepted my score. Dylan beamed at his, and tittuped into the dining hall in a lively and exaggerated manner, as actors tended to do when on stage. The line to get our food was not too long, and we sat at a table facing the windows.

"Gary, you are too serious," Dylan said, breaking the silence.

"The girls are only having fun. This was just a sport and it was a game. And they only did this as part of their pledge week for the sororities, anyway. Besides, we guys do this all the time," Dylan reminded me.

"We always rated the girls from one to ten even when it was not pledge week. This was just fun, it is only a game," Dylan chuckled and said, "It's a sport, it's entertainment, it's only done in fun."

"That's easy for you to say, all your scores blew completely off the chart."

"This was just fun, a game, a sport," Dylan repeated to convince me, as he swallowed down almost the entire plate of spaghetti in one gulp.

"Uhm, I guess so."

But Dylan had never been in a police lineup. He never had the experience of being told to face forward, turn to the left, turn to the right. "You, number three, step forward."

But for that matter, neither had I. I had only imagined Sam going through that procedure after being arrested for breaking car windows outside the community center. He was in jail for vagrancy and breach of peace. But, he had said that he was in a line up for the investigation of some other crimes that had happened. I vowed to avoid going through any procedure like that in my life. Therefore, whether this happened in a jail lock up, or on a red bricked path into a dining hall on a bucolic campus was not really important to me. I did not want to live that experience, and now it felt like I was going through what I vowed I would not.

The sun was still streaming through the large windows into the Annex, the newer part of the dining hall. I loved looking out the glass windows to see the outside trees and shrubs. The windows were majestic and took up one side of the wall, going from the floor to ceiling. The glass met the ceiling at the top and formed a sharp "V" as an arrow would have. It pointed straight up to the sky. In this room when the sunlight streamed in, and you connected with the wide open space and sky, you felt one with the universe. It only meant you should aspire to be free, moving onwards and upwards. But the girls reminded me that there was another reality. That there was also the reality of being grounded yet scrutinized, bound, tethered.

I looked through the clear glass and up into the sky to catch the last rays of sunlight before the night would fall and bring out the stars, planets, and moon. Ah, I loved the sun. I grinned and pushed the spaghetti away from me towards Dylan. He excitedly plowed into the second plate of spaghetti and meatballs, and gobbled half the plate down in one swallow.

"Yes, you can have another one of the dining hall's special meals," I thought.

On the weekend, I was sitting with some other friends watching a football game. We sometimes lull ourselves into believing that we are not affected by our experiences, and that it is simple enough to pick ourselves up, and brush ourselves off. But, though that is our intent, it usually takes a concerted effort to recover from the fall, perceived or real. My scores flashed through my mind again. I vigorously rubbed my eyes to make the memory go away. Maybe, I was also muttering something to myself, as Carla, who had been intent on the game's action, broke the silence.

"Why are your eyes closed? Why aren't you watching the football game?" they both asked. "What's up with you anyway?"

"Oh, my contacts are jammed, I had to close my eyes," I said to misinform them. I pretended that I was trying to flick the contact lens back in place by blinking multiple times. I said no more, feigning concentration on getting them back in place on my eyeballs. Harrison and Carla realized that I had no intention of answering the "What's up with you anyway?" question, and certainly not as fast as they wanted. Therefore, they decided to ignore me and returned to watch the football game that was being played on the field.

Of course, I was going to ignore their question. I needed to focus and get my eyes right. I could not see where I was going. My vision was clouded. Who can think, plan, and create without a vision. No mission. No strategy. I decided not to respond. Similar to a position that we may take when hurt, I retreated to pout, to be defiant. I was not going to answer them. I would not answer until I was good and ready. Furthermore, I needed my eyes not to be red and bloodshot. Carla and Harrison paid no attention to me and locked their eyes onto the action on the football field. They were sports fanatics and were used to sitting at sporting events on hard bleachers. They sat forward and leaned even more to get a better look at the field. They were used to everything. Nothing seemed to faze them. They looked at the players on the football field who were sacking and tossing and tackling their opponents to the ground. They sat on that bench, ignored me some more, and would not move their eyes off the field. At least they had vision and could see. I mostly felt that my own vision was cloudy.

When I realized that I needed their feedback, and that defiance would get me nowhere, I interrupted them. I asked, "Are my eyes blood shot red?"

Harrison laughed.

"Of course they are. Blood red and shot," Harrison mocked. "They look like a hot mess," Harrison said.

Harrison was always blunt and to the point. He was not the type to tell you what you wanted to hear. If you didn't want to hear the truth, or if you were not ready to hear it, he was the last person you wanted to talk to. He came at you point blank with no sugar coating. Since, I had interrupted them looking at the football game, they both turned away again. Harrison turned to concentrate on the football game that was being played on the field. Carla stared blankly at her feet.

"Yeah? Who cares if your eyes are red? Everyone will just think that you smoked something," Harrison said.

"Hah. Hah. That would be a first for you," Harrison laughed.

"Yeah, that would be a first," Carla chimed in.

"Once bitten, twice shy," I thought. I had lived with the paranoia of having my eyes look like Sam's had ever since Sam came home from the hospital with bandages on both eyes. His eyes were blood shot red. He could not see for about a week. How could I ever tell my friends about this paranoia, when I had never even mention Sam and what he had gone through? How could I do it and make them understand what that was like? When could I tell them what it was like seeing him struggle and what life was like living with him?

fear, hypo- chondria secrets

Sleepwalking

"Hey, wake up. It's your turn to wake us up in thirty minutes. We've got to finish reading through the two hundred pages before class starts at eight o'clock in the morning," I said.

"Well, you know that's not going to happen. We will never finish all of this by then. Why don't we just divide and conquer. I will read the first fifty pages. Nina can read the next fifty, and Julia the next fifty, and you can read the remainder. When we have read our parts then we can summarize it and tell each other what's the most important issue," Leo said.

"Yeah, that should do."

"How do I even know that you will correctly distill the most important stuff?" I asked.

"What if you are too sleepy and you give me the wrong information?"

"Well, you just have to trust me," Leo responded.

"Huh? There are three things that gets my eyebrows to twitching and raises my radar," Nina chimed in to say.

"What's that?" Julia asked.

"Trust me, I love you, and I am good for it," Nina said.

"Why's that?" Julia asked.

"First, let's take the first one, "I love you,"" Nina said.

"It rolls too easily off people's lips. First, you don't even know me. You met me yesterday. How can you love me? What does it mean? What do you mean, love, what does that look like? Or people say that when they want your physical body to use for a period, to satisfy some physical need that they have."

"*Nyet.* I don't buy it," Nina said. "In the twinkling of an eye once they have gotten what they came for, you are tossed in the garbage heap."

"The next thing is, "I am good for it," you know," Nina said.

"Yes, I know about that one too," I said.

"Folks are always coming to you to say, "lend me this and lend me that," Nina added.

"You know very well that lend me means "give me". And they know very well that they have no intention to give you back that money lent. Yeah, I am good for it for Friday."

"Yeah, right!" Nina scornfully said.

"Friday will come and they start to avoid you. The next Friday will come and nothing. No call, no nothing. The next time they see you, they look straight at you and not even say, Nina, I have not forgotten about that thing. Nothing."

"So, I trust you, I am good for it, I love you. No, no, no!" Nina screamed.

"Well, forget the other one," Leo said. "Nina, you are too young to be so cynical. Anyway, forget the other one, let's get back to work."

"Well, that's just it," Nina said.

"What is just it?" Julia asked.

Leo protested. "But, we have all these pages to read. We need to pass these tests. We cannot read all this information tonight. Now it is two hundred pages. Tomorrow it is another two hundred. This is not going to go away."

"That's why I don't like the last one," Nina said.

"You know it too, Gary and Julia. Trust me," Nina said. "You have to trust me."

"That gets my goad a-going."

"So guess what, guys, you have to trust me. You have to trust that I am going to stay awake and read and comprehend and interpret and give you the correct information."

"You just have to trust. You just have to have faith and trust."

"No, I don't buy it," Nina said. "Why should I trust you? You have to work at getting my trust. I am not going to trust you blindly. And if you start the conversation with saying trust me, that's a red flag for me," Nina said.

"Nina, sometimes, you just have to trust. You can't live a life full of cynicism and sarcasm. Sometimes, you have to blindly trust and hope that is the right decision," Julia said.

"Like now. You have to trust me that I will stay awake, read, and interpret the material correctly, and summarize it clearly and succinctly for you. This is too much for one person to do by themselves. You have to trust, give up some control. That is how we all get through this. If you don't, we all are unnecessarily stressed and increase our individual risk of failing. You have to trust us."

"I guess you are right," Nina conceded. "But, I am watching you. One false move and that's it."

"Look," I said. "Let's trust each other. And right now, it is my turn to keep watch. You guys have thirty minutes each to take a nap and then I will wake you up. I don't intend in staying up all night without not even an ounce of shut eye. I am not Sam," I said.

"What about Sam?" Leo asked.

"Oh, nothing," I said.

It was not unusual at times for Sam to stay up for two to three nights at a time. He would be agitated and paced the floor all night long. How he could remain so wired, awake, and still stand up after that was remarkable. Sometimes, he would talk. Sometimes, he would not. I could not run on fumes like that. And I also know that doing so was not healthy.

In medical school the perpetual lack of sleep was an unwelcomed necessity. We had lots to read. Working and studying alone did not make much sense. If you did that, the burn-out rate was high.

I could not function while sleepwalking. Nina was right and she was wrong. We had to trust that the persons we gave our trust to had our best interests at heart. But, to not trust at all only meant carrying an unbearable burden. One of the things I learned in medical school is to know your strengths and to know your weaknesses. You had to know when to ask for help. Being a hero was not always a good idea and being mature and asking for help was not a sign of weakness. It was a sign of common sense and asking for help to fill in gaps in information and asking where to go for help.

Helter Skelter Broken Pieces

At the end of the first year of medical school, I came home but, in one week I was to go to New York City to work in the city morgue for the rest of the summer. I had gotten a summer job there to work in one of the busiest morgues in the world.

I worked with a pathologist who was interested in studying the anatomy and brain chemistry of people who had committed suicide. I would go into work early in the morning and get out by 3 p.m. in the afternoon. The morgue was in the basement, and it was cold and damp. The morgue attendants were skillful with their saws, and respectful of the persons entrusted in their care. They always said never to forget that this was someone's loved one, mother, father, sister, brother, lover, friend. Somewhere there was someone grieving and never to forget that.

The cold air down there chilled my bones, and at the end of my shift I was glad to get back out to the clean air, at least New York City clean. In comparison to the chemically laced, disinfected, air that I breathed there for the eight hours in the basement, I welcomed the car-exhausted, people-rebreathed, building-trapped air that permeated the city. I happily sucked it into my lungs to exchange the stagnant one that I was forced to inhale in a hall filled with steel tables and matching containers.

That summer, Sam had continued to act strangely. He had begun to hear voices and see things. He was not working and spent a lot of time in his room by himself. Everything was going downhill fast. He started a job working at the airport and in one day he had quit. He claimed that the boss asked him to do something and he thought he spoke to him with the wrong tone of voice.

"What tone of voice was that?"

"He said that I should go do the job that I was hired to do."

"Well, that's not a tone of voice," Esther said. "You were hired to do a job. They are not going to pay you for doing nothing."

And so the spiral downwards into nothingness began. Subsequently, alcohol became the problem and him being drunk all day. It was this beer then that beer, every day, all day. I supposed the alcohol was medication to calm the voices in this head and replace the dead people he was seeing.

There was not a day that I was not glad to get away to go to New York, even if it meant working in the morgue. I was starting to feel numb and this place of cold, dampness, and steel was as good as any to keep me company. But, I had only exchanged the Artic for the Antarctic. I had moved from dealing with an odd brother to working with doctors who were also a different bunch. Working with the pathologist, I was glad my job was only to help him as he did his dissections for the autopsies. I did not want to touch any part of the brain even though I had gloves on. We always got the interesting cases. He was talkative and would tell me all the different stories about how that person came to be in the morgue. I didn't want to know why or how they got there then. Now, I appreciate the many paths that each person had taken to get to that place in their lives. I was too young then to see the connections of all the things in our lives and the common bonds that we share.

False Friends

I don't know how I would have gotten through college or medical school without the friends that pulled me through. We all crave that need for friendship to sustain us in all our activities. Yet, sometimes it can become hard to tell friend from foe.

Sam too had many friends. When his mind was somewhat intact he was the life of the party. He told the funniest jokes, made the weirdest connections between things, remembered things way back from the past long after you had forgotten them. He talked a lot, and laughed a lot, and people held their stomachs, laughing out loud saying, "You're out of your mind!"

He got in your face and talked, and commented about why you wore that pants or shirt or dress or earrings or watch, and linked it to something he saw on the streets, in jail or in a movie. Sometimes the connections made sense, most often they did not, but they were interesting none-the-less. The connections made you pause to think. The friends laughed and held their bellies in to prevent from exploding, and could not stop laughing. Sometimes I think that is why he hated the medications because they kept that edgy side at bay.

Once, in between jail and the long psychiatric hospitalizations, to get Sam off the streets he was living in an apartment. It was small, but it was his place and somewhere to be out of the cold. Esther had to co-sign the lease for the apartment. Like our need for friendship, we all seek independence. Sam was living alone, and the freedom was good at first.

Soon after that though, Sam stopped taking his medications. When you have lots of friends, choosing those who have your best interest at heart can be hard. In addition, each one may not know your particular situation; therefore, they cannot tell you that what is good for the goose may not be good for the gander. They may not know what your breaking points are, and what you can cope with. In no time Sam was not even in the apartment much. He was starting to walk the streets and the spiral down began. Since he was hardly there, the false friends took over the apartment.

Esther knocked on the door and it was opened by some strange type.

"Where is Sam?" she asked.

"Oh, he is not here."

Esther stood there shocked while the smell of marijuana assaulted her nose and the stench of days-old alcohol choked her. The filth of the apartment disgusted her, as there were empty beer cans, rum bottles, vodka carafes, old newspapers, and cigarette butts everywhere. Dirty laundry was on the floor, dirty dishes were piled in the sink, and dirt, dust, and grime was everywhere.

"How could this happen in one week, two weeks tops?"

Esther walked out of the apartment and slammed the door shut.

"I have to find Sam. This is foolish. At this rate if something is not done Sam will be the death of me."

"They have to take this apartment back. I cannot deal with this. No. And on top of that I am liable for the rest of the lease if he breaks it? Is he for real?"

"They know Sam is sick. Who really needs friends like that?" she asked.

CHAPTER 7

BURNING THE
MIDNIGHT OIL

I did not understand what the problem was in Room 15, and most of the information about why the man was in the emergency room was not filled in by the nurse. Why was the man here today? Usually when that happened it was because it was a very personal problem, and the patient did not want to tell the triage nurse. In that case, the nurse would decide to let him explain everything to the doctor. It was better that way, to not make the patient uncomfortable at the beginning of the emergency room experience.

The patient, a male in his mid-thirties, was in the emergency room at midnight. The triage nurse had simply recorded "general symptoms." I took note of the usual readings that the nurse made, and that the man had allowed, and they were all normal.

"Why is he here with general complaints in the middle of the night? In a couple of hours I would think he should be at work. Did he not have a primary care doctor to go to?" I asked myself. I rapped on the room door, stepped into the room, and closed the door behind me.

"Hi, I am Dr. Gary," I said and pulled my badge forward so that he could read my name.

"What's your name, sir?"

"Oh, me, what's my name?"

I looked around the room. He and I were the only persons there. I had just told him my name. There was no one else in the room, and it should be obvious that I was speaking to him. Was someone else here that I could not see? I was used to living with that. I smiled and was on the verge of laughing out loud. Invisible people were everywhere so you can't be too sure. I wanted to laugh from the memory, but, professionalism was the golden rule. I suppressed the urge to laugh out loud and asked him to confirm his name. I knew it should be Mr. Gardener, as that was who the patient list had noted to be in Room 15. But, I wanted him to tell me his name, and then I would look at his name tag on his wrist to confirm that I was speaking to the correct person.

"Yes, sir, what's your name?"

"Oh, Kent Gardener."

"Mr. Gardener, I am Dr. Gary, the emergency room doctor." I reached out and shook his right hand.

"May I look at your name tag that the registration clerk put on your wrist?"

"Sure."

He stuck out his left wrist for me to read his name, and the tag also had his date of birth and the current date on it. It also had a scanning barcode. The nurses could verify his identity with a portable scanner, and they would scan the barcode if they gave him any medications. The name tag and barcode were also used if he had to get any other examinations, laboratory tests, X-Rays or CAT scans. We used it to make sure the right patient got the right treatment. The name tag on his left wrist was the same as the name that he told me.

"Ok, Mr. Gardener, what's wrong that brings you to the emergency room tonight?"

"Well, I have a problem."

He was sitting on the bed with both legs dangling over the edge. He had not undressed for an exam. I was sure that Brian, the nurse assigned to these rooms tonight, had told him to at least take his shirt off and put on the hospital gown. The hospital gown still lay neatly folded at his side and he had not touched it. I interpreted that to mean that he came to the emergency room, not necessarily for an examination, but for advice. It must be pretty serious for him to be out of his bed at this time of night.

"What's the problem?"

I moved to sit on the chair that was in the room because I did not want to stand over him. That would give him the impression that I was in a rush. It would appear that I did not want to listen to the problem that brought him to emergency room. I turned the chair on its swivel several times to get the chair and the bed to be at the same level. When I sat down in the chair I wanted to be at eye level with him as we spoke. After I was comfortable that the three swivels would leave both of us at a similar level in a sitting position, I stopped turning the chair and sat down. I sat down and was proud that I had judged the turns correctly. It had only taken three turns to sufficiently bring the chair and the bed to the same height.

"Well, I was sick last week."

I did not interrupt him and I looked at him to encourage him to continue speaking.

"I was very sick last week," he continued. "I had like a headache, fever, and chills."

"You know, I like, had the flu. My muscles were achy, very achy. I had a sore throat and like a cold," he kept going on. "Oh, I had a rash on my face and chest too."

I sat there and just let him talk. I knew that he would eventually come around to say what was really on his mind.

"I had a high fever," he said again. "But in a day or two, it was gone. The flu and all the symptoms went away in a day or two. You know, I don't get sick."

I guess he was trying to convince me that he doesn't get sick. Well, I don't know that you don't get sick, I thought to myself. I just met you, and I am not your primary care doctor, therefore, I would not really know that you don't get sick. But, you are right. You appear as if you are fairly healthy. You are properly clothed for the weather. You seem to have access to food and are well nourished. It appears that you take care of your physical body.

You probably do some type of exercise to stay in physical shape. Your speech is clear and coherent. You know where you are, and I assume you know the time. You know your name because you told me so. As to your current mental or emotional state, I would have to ask you some more questions. I could observe your behaviors to try to figure out what is going on. But, I don't know that you don't get sick. I wouldn't "know" unless you told me.

"But, you said there was a problem."

"Yes."

"I think that you just said that. One week ago, you were sick for about two to three days? Is that right?"

"Yes."

"And that you were having a fever, chills, sore throat, a rash, muscles aches and pains, and a headache, right?"

"Yes. Oh, I had a dry cough too. But, it all went away after two to three days. You see, I never get sick."

"Ok," I said. "Did you have other symptoms, other problems? For example, did you have nausea, vomiting or diarrhea?"

"No."

"With the headache, was your neck stiff? What about your vision, was it blurry? Did you have any problems with your memory?"

"No."

"Did anyone tell you that you seemed confused when you had the fever and the headache?" I asked.

It did not sound as if he had meningitis, an inflammation of the lining of the brain. With meningitis, other symptoms might have been neck stiffness, fever, confusion, nausea, and maybe vomiting. He had recovered too quickly based on what he was saying, so any type of meningitis, viral or bacterial was extremely unlikely.

"And the rash is now gone?"

"Yes."

"Do you have any medical problems? Are you seeing a doctor for any reason?" I said, rephrasing the question.

Maybe he did not understand what I was asking. Did he know if he had any medical problems? Maybe he had not been to a doctor. So he could have a medical problem and not know it.

"What I mean is your doctor treating you for something, like diabetes, asthma, or high blood pressure? Any problems like that?"

"Do you take any medications on a regular basis? Anything prescribed by a doctor? Or are you taking anything over counter?" I asked. "Do you have any allergies?"

"No, none of that."

"Have you traveled anywhere? Have you been outside of the state or outside the country? Have you been anywhere?"

"No."

"Do you have a doctor that you see regularly, at some time or another?"

"Well, yeah. I have one assigned by my insurance company. The doctor's name is on the card. But, to tell you the truth, Doc, I have never gone to see him."

"Did you call him for an appointment? Did you call to tell him what was going on over the last couple of days, or last week?"

"No, no. I did not call him. But, I was too worried to go there anyway. Do you think I have something?" he asked.

"I mean, do you think I could have caught something?" he asked again. He was asking now with more concern in his voice. He was worried about something. What was it?

Okay, I thought. He is worried about something. Where is his line of questioning going? He is in the emergency room in the middle of the night to talk to a doctor about something that was on his mind. He did not feel that he could wait and make an appointment with his doctor. It wasn't a true emergency in the truest sense of the word. He was not about to lose his life or limb. He did not have chest pain, belly pains or a headache. If he had waited to see his doctor, any doctor in the morning, he was not going to die, right? At least, it did not seem that way to me. What was really up with all this?

"Can you check my blood pressure and make sure I am Okay?" he asked.

"Sure. I will check it again for you. But, do you mind if I ask you some more questions first?"

"No, I am all ears."

"Mr. Gardener, from what you told me, it sounds as if you had a viral syndrome last week. A syndrome means that you had some symptoms or complaints and a cluster of signs or problems. You were sick for only a short period."

"There are a couple of things that come to my mind that could do that. But I have some more questions for you. Do you mind if I ask you some more questions?"

He nodded his approval.

"What I am going to ask you are some very personal questions. Is that okay with you?" I asked again.

"I don't know what your experience has been like with other doctors or your health care provider. So, don't get surprised by what I am going to ask you. I am only here to help and understand what the next steps are. I do not think that you want me to just do random tests without having an idea of what we are looking for," I said.

I thought—you did not want to tell the nurse what was the real concern that brought you to the emergency room at mid-night. You did not undress and you have made it a point to say that you are never sick. You had a viral illness last week. You now feel better, but something else was on your mind.

"Are you sexually active?"

"Yes, I am in a relationship."

"Do you have one or more than one partner?"

"Well, I am married."

"Okay, you are married," I said and confirmed that I had heard him on that one. But, I pressed on anyway with my questions.

"Are you monogamous, meaning, do you have only one partner?" I asked again to clarify the question.

"Well, you can't tell my wife," he said.

What? I can't tell your wife that you are married? Doesn't your wife know that you are married? Are you not married to her? Huh, I thought, well, who exactly is your wife, I don't think I know her, do I?

"Don't tell your wife what?"

"Well, I slept with another woman. I met her at a bar about three weeks ago."

"Mr. Gardener, I would not tell your wife that unless you gave me permission to do so."

"Besides, there is the issue of patient privacy and confidentiality. I would not be allowed to give your wife that information without your consent. You would have to tell me that you agree and give permission for me to tell her. That means, even with your medical conditions, you would have to give me verbal and written permission for me to tell her what you tell me."

"I had never done that before. You know, cheated on my wife. I used a condom but I am not sure that I really protected myself. And who knows? Condoms break, right? I don't know why I did that. Cheated, I mean. Now, I need to make sure that I did not catch anything and worse yet give something to my wife. I should never have done that. I don't know what I was thinking. I was not thinking," he said.

"Mr. Gardener, I am not here to judge you. But, I can give you information that is useful. I will also give you my advice. I can also tell you where you may get other information and how to get it," I said.

"Yeah, that's why I am here. What should I do, Doc?"

"If you had an encounter where you did not use safe sex practices, you are at risk of getting a sexually transmitted infection, or STI. You are probably used to hear people saying STD for short. The STDs that you may have been exposed to are, HIV, the virus that causes AIDS, gonorrhea, syphilis, chlamydia, herpes, among others. I don't mean to scare you."

"At the point when you first become infected with HIV, you might have something that seems like a viral illness. You may feel like you got the "flu." It could be similar to the problems that you had."

"You may get a fever, chills, muscle aches and pain, sore throat, and a headache. You may even have a cough and what we call an upper respiratory infection."

"The information that you had these complaints after you had sex would make me suggest that you get an HIV test. I also recommend that you test for the other STDs that I talked about. These are herpes, syphilis, gonorrhea, and chlamydia. Some of these tests are blood tests. Some of them are test that we do on a sample of your urine," I said, pausing so that he could follow what I was saying.

"Yes, well that's why I came in tonight. I really want you to test me for HIV. I did not want to tell the nurses that when I came in to the emergency department. But that's really why I am here. I could not sleep another night without getting that test done I have not been able to sleep well just thinking about it. What if I picked up something?" he asked.

"Well, there are a couple of steps that we must go through. I can help you as much as I can tonight and then I will need to refer you to either your doctor, or to the City's Health Department for some of the other tests. At the City's Health Department, you can get your HIV testing done confidentially. That means you can get the test done with your information protected."

"You will be counseled about what it means to get the HIV test. They will tell you what the test results mean. If the test is negative, you should repeat the test in six months. We do that to make sure that from that last time you had sex, you did not become infected. On that first test it may have been too early to tell if you were infected with the HIV virus."

"So, again, first we explain what the HIV test means. We tell you what it means to have a negative result or a positive result. We also tell you what the next steps are based on the result of your test," I said.

"Can you do the test tonight?"

"Well, no, not quite. At the present time, this emergency room only tests for HIV if an employee is exposed to blood or body fluids. We do not routinely test anyone who comes into the emergency room for an HIV test, as you have done. In addition to all of that, it is important that we can contact you to tell you the results of the test. We would need to find you to give you all the necessary information, and make sure that you have a health care provider that you can see to take care of you once you are tested. One of the best places to get free testing is the City's Health Department. They are open at eight o'clock in the morning, Monday to Friday. The test is free and it is confidential. They will tell you about the test. They will make sure that they can find you to give you the test results. They will also make sure that you have a health care provider that you can see to take care of you, no matter if the test is positive or negative. If the test comes back positive, they will also help in finding the persons that you had sex with. That way, if you did not feel comfortable with telling that person yourself, they can contact them. They can reach them and tell them that a partner tested positive and encourage them to get tested so that they can know their status."

"That's a lot of information all at once. Do you have any questions so far?" I asked.

"No. Well it's almost one o'clock in the morning. I do not have to go to work until 3 p.m. today. So, I can get the test when they open at eight o'clock in the morning."

"Yes," I said, "that would be the best thing for you to do."

"Mr. Gardener, it is important for anyone who has ever been sexually active to know their status. If you have had sex once, or whether it is more than once, it is important to know your status."

"If you know your status, you can protect yourself and others, and reduce your risks of getting HIV infection, or giving it to someone else," I said. "In fact, the Centers for Disease Control, the CDC, recommend routine HIV screening for all patients, ages thirteen to sixty-four years old. So, it is something our doctors should recommend so that we all know our status."

"You may also want to know that having certain sexually transmitted diseases increases the chance of getting infected with HIV."

"And if you have HIV and other STDs, there is a greater chance of spreading HIV to others. I know that you said that you have been healthy all your life. Let's try to keep it that way."

"But some problems like substance use and abuse, including injection drug use, mental health problems, childhood sexual abuse, and other emotional stress may make it difficult for people to protect themselves and their partners."

"If you are going through some of these emotional stressors, it may make it harder to protect yourself and your partners from these STDs," I said.

"So, are you saying that if I have these emotional conditions or stress, I am going to get these infections?"

"No, I am not saying that at all. Any sexually active person can be exposed to sexually transmitted infections, STIs or STDS."

"However, when you are going through emotional stress, you are at increased risk because you may be in a relationship where you may be more vulnerable to partner pressures."

"When you are stressed you may take chances that you would otherwise not take. It increases risky behaviors."

"One of the things that we should do is to break the silence, and to increase awareness about HIV and AIDS, so that friends, family, co-workers, and many others are informed. There are no boundaries now with HIV, they have all been crossed."

"I think we should talk about it more and educate each other to protect each other. So, tonight, here's what I am thinking. Let me know what you think?" I asked.

"Okay."

"I think it is important for us to know our HIV status."

"I recommend that you get tested for all the infections I mentioned, HIV, gonorrhea, syphilis, chlamydia, and herpes."

"The City's Health Department opens at eight o'clock. You may get all your tests for free there and it is confidential. Remember, you will have to go through the counseling about what the test results mean. And it is important for them to see you again to go over your test results. So give them the right phone number and address so that they can reach you."

"Does that make any sense?"

"Yes, it does."

"I will go and get all the tests done in the morning."

"Okay."

"Here is my card with my name and telephone number on it."

"If you have any problems about getting it done, please feel free to call me, and I will help you get to the place that you are comfortable getting the tests done."

"I can call you for more information if needed?"

"Of course, you can."

"All the doctors here have business cards with our names on it. That way you know who treated you, and you can call us if you have questions."

"But, above all this, I recommend that you call your primary care doctor and make an appointment."

"There are many reasons to have a regular health care provider. We call that a medical home. A medical home is like home. It is a place where the providers know you and can take care of you. They can make the referrals that you need, and do the tests that are needed. They can do all the prevention screens and tests that you need. You will get to know them and they will get to know you, like family."

"What about my wife, what should I tell her?"

"Well, I think that is more complicated."

"You may want to speak to a counselor, by yourself, or together with your wife. Talking to a counselor may help you think about and explain some of the reasons that led you to have an encounter with someone else who was not your partner."

"I will give you a list of counselors that you may call, if you would like."

"Yes, thanks, Doc."

"Give me the list so I can call. I think I will need help in telling her, but I know that I must do that."

"Is there anything else tonight?"

"No. I am glad I came in tonight."

"So am I, Mr. Gardener."

"Okay. So, here are the places, addresses, and phone numbers where you can get all your tests done. So, see that you go in the morning." I handed the list to him and he shook my hand.

"I am glad you came into the emergency room tonight," I repeated to reassure him.

"Yes, so am I," he said.

CHAPTER 8

TREE TRUNKS

S am was trying to sit in the front passenger seat of the car. He went in
head first with half of his body parallel to the seat. His left knee rested
on the seat, and the right one was sticking out the open car door. I
stood there staring, trying to figure out what contortions he would need to
make to get seated properly in the car. I judged that there was no way for him
to get seated in the car given the way he had entered head first.

He should be sober by now after last night's fiasco. He put his sneakers on
and he walked out the house without his cane. He really needed that cane for
balance. He had degenerative arthritis in both knees—the right knee being
worse than the left. He developed these conditions from years of overuse of
unnecessarily walking long distances. Sometimes, rather than taking a bus,
he walked from one end of the city to the other end. He aimlessly wandered
with no destination, and seldom stopped to rest.

Previously, he walked the five miles from the mental health center to the
center of downtown. Then he stood downtown for several hours and then
walked all the way back to the assisted living center. When Charlie, one of
the attendants, called me to take a look at his legs, I was horrified. Sam's legs

looked like tree trunks, and the swelling went all the way up to his groin. I could not distinguish the knee from the rest of the leg. The ankles and foot were severely swollen, red, and painful. The soles of the feet were blistering. The ankles I recognized. They looked like Gasterre's ankles. All the natural contour of the ankles and legs were distorted, and Sam wobbled when he stood to stand or to walk.

Oh, God, I thought, why did Sam do that? Why did he not stop and sit? He could have called me. He could have called the assisted living center. He probably had my cell phone number and Charlie's number written on a piece of paper somewhere in his pocket. I usually had that written on a card or paper that he kept. I kicked myself for not getting him the name tag with the contact numbers that I promised I would get and put around his wrist or neck. The Army calls these dog tags. I hated the term dog tags, but I really needed Sam to have one to wear for identification. His wallet could get stolen. Or who knows? More often than not, he tossed the wallet away anyway.

He should have tried to call somebody. For several weeks after that episode, Sam's legs were so swollen that he waddled down the hallway, and it took him forever to move an inch. He refused to use a wheel chair; that would have been the best option to move around. We got him a cane and he preferred to use that. But truth be told, the cane did not really help either. The leg swelling was so severe that only time would heal them. When I saw his legs so swollen, I had insisted that we go to the emergency room to get an ultrasound to make sure there were no clots in his legs. There were no clots, and we were discharged from the emergency room with instructions for him to raise his legs above heart level.

Well, he hardly ever did as he was told. At night he would pace in his room and in the halls. He would go back and forth. It was if he were an infantry who was given marching orders and was not told when to stop. If his mind told him to stand, walk, and pace, neither swelling, pain or blistering would stop him. Short of restraining him in bed, there was probably no way for me to get him to stay still. There was always the option of giving him a sedative so that he would sleep, or adjusting his other medications. But, for the leg swelling at least, there were very few options. Only watchful waiting and time would make a difference.

Sam had walked and paced and stood in one place unnecessarily so many times before that the knee joints were worn out. The body is like a car, like a machine. If you took care of the car and took it for regular checkups, changing the sparks and oils and wheels, and whatever else is changeable, it may last you a very long time. But, if you mistreated the car, used and abused it and never did any preventive care, it may not last you a very long time. With modern medicine, you could replace joints and an organ or two. But modern science is still very far away from replacing the entire chassis, or the engine, or the brain.

Therefore, now, I was watching in confusion as Sam contorted himself trying to figure out how he would get himself into the front seat.

"Sam, you will never get into the car seat doing that. Why don't you start over? Get out of the car. Stand up first. Put your bottom on the front seat with your legs still on the ground. Ease yourself into the front seat, and use the handle above the door to help you in. Get your left foot in first. After you do that, I can help you get your right leg in."

He turned and looked at me. Maybe he had forgotten that he was getting into a car seat and not into another dark tunnel.

Sam smiled saying, "Oh, I knew that."

I looked at my watch and moved forward to help him get his right leg into the car.

"Look, Sam," I said. "I need to drop you off at the assisted living center. I have work at 2 p.m. today. I am running late already with errands. Later on today, if I get a minute at work, I will call you. I also need to speak to Marlon or Charlie. I need to figure out what to do."

I started the car and reversed from the driveway. The way to the assisted living center today seemed to take forever and I simply had no time to lose.

"Trees. Tree trunks. Hills. Mountains. Move. Get out of my way today for once, please" I begged.

Legs

I hated that buzz and it always started that way. The public announcement system had a grating noise like chalk striking a blackboard. When the noise stopped, I paused to hear what the announcement was.

"Trauma Team, STAT, to the Trauma Room, Trauma Team, STAT, to the Trauma Room."

"Gosh," I said, "is that the same one or another one? I just had a full trauma less than five minutes ago. What is going on out there today?"

Well, I knew what was going on. There was a concert in the city today. That usually meant more people and more cars and we were busier than normal. I wished it to be as with most concerts. We got the drunken college students who the paramedics extracted from the mosh pit for their own safety, and brought them to the emergency room for evaluation. Our mantra in the emergency room was safety first. If you could not keep the patient or yourself safe, there would be little else you could accomplish medically. Until you did that, all work was at a standstill.

"Trauma Team, STAT, to the Trauma Room, Trauma Team, STAT, to the Trauma Room!"

All the pagers and phones were ringing, and the residents and other doctors who had lingered from the prior full trauma pressed the keys to stop them from beeping.

"Trauma Team, STAT, to the Trauma Room, Trauma Team, STAT, to the Trauma Room!" the operator said for the third time.

"What is it?" I asked Magdalene—who preferred to be called Lena—the nurse now in charge. She came into the Trauma Room to get the trauma paperwork ready.

"It is a young woman. She was hit by a train," Lena said somberly.

"How, where, why, when? What happened?"

"I don't really know," Lena said. "But the paramedics are on scene. They have already "tubed" her but I am not sure they got her blood pressure back. I think she must be in a shock state. They said they are, like, two minutes out."

We prepared and quickly gowned, gloved, and masked to be ready when they arrived. Suddenly, Howard, the paramedic, barged into the trauma room with the other members of his crew. He immediately started to talk to give us his report.

"We found this young woman on the train tracks," Howard said. His speech was crisp but pressured. He tried to remain calm, but it was difficult to do so.

We had become too numb by seeing or hearing that someone was injured. Violence was all around us. It was everywhere, in the movies, on television, or at home. We started to think that this was a normal part of life. But, from birth to the grave, we should be preventing injuries. Injuries are not accidents and most, if not all of them, can be prevented. In the pediatrician's office, the health care provider advises parents how to keep their children free from injuries. Having a home that is safe for a child so that he or she is not injured was important. Older adults in their homes should also be concerned about injuries from falls. Safety was first—in the home, in school, at work, or on the road—wherever we were.

Whether Sam was floridly psychotic or not, I think about keeping him safe all the time. I needed him safe to not injure himself, or to injure others. Often, while working in the emergency room or elsewhere, health care providers are exposed to actual, potential or a threat of violence. We learn to be extremely observant of behaviors and our surroundings. Objects that seem harmless, belts and buckles, and draw strings from pants, may be used as weapons. If the patient appears to have a behavioral or mental health condition, awareness and observation by the provider is essential to keep the patient and the provider safe. We remove all contrabands, sharps, razors, knives, guns, lighters, belts, you name it.

Safety was first for all patients, but even more so with the psychotic patient. The provider needed to watch for subtle signs of agitation. We were careful not to overstimulate the patient. We did not make direct eye contact unnecessarily and we kept a submissive pose. Our voice was calm and reassuring. We did not put our bodies in such a way as if to obstruct or prevent the patient's exit or block their way. If we needed reinforcement to subdue a patient, then we called on security and others to assist.

"Yah," Howard said now more slowly, and in less of a rush.

"We found her on the train tracks."

"The train ran over both legs. I don't think the train driver even saw her, or even if he had any time to stop."

"We do not know if she fell, but she was on her back. There did not appear to be any injuries above the knees, as her head, chest, and belly did not show any other signs of trauma."

"She was in shock and unconscious. We intubated her on the scene and placed two large bore IVs in each upper arm. I am not sure if she was drinking or not."

"Her blood pressure was low and she was barely breathing. When we "tubed" her she hardly responded to us. Her skin was cold and clammy. We wrapped her legs in sterile towels, did what we could and got here as fast as possible."

"She is in shock," Howard said.

"Yes, looks that way," I said. "She has practically bled out."

Four doctors and nurses jumped into action working at the bed side and stationing at each limb. I was at the head to manage the airway. We quickly placed her on the monitor so that we could all see the vital signs, the blood pressure, heart rate, and oxygen level. Someone took her temperature, and Lena put all of that information on the trauma flow sheet.

"We need the operating room ready, blood, antibiotics, fluids, now," Luke said.

"Lena, call Vascular and Orthopedics, we need them to meet us in the operating room now," Dr. Luke Jones said.

"Let's get the initial X-Rays here of the neck, chest, and pelvis to be sure there are no other injuries to the neck, lungs, and pelvis," I said.

Luke pulled over the portable ultrasound machine to quickly scan the heart, lungs, liver, kidney, spleen, and bladder. Satisfied that the portable X-Rays showed no other injuries, and that the ultrasound showed no other organs injured or rupture, we started the next steps.

"Great, we are off to the operating room," Luke said as he and his team dashed with the patient and the stretcher down the hallway to the short elevator ride to the operating room.

"Let me know how things work out," I said.

"We will let the police confirm her identity and reach her family."

Safety was the essential step to prevent the violence and stop all these injuries. What did we have to do to get there?

Straightjacket

It was seven o'clock in the morning and therefore all the clients had to leave the homeless shelter for the day. They were not allowed to come back into the building until five o'clock in the evening. Some of the clients had jobs and went to work for the day. Others had some place to go to sit for the day. Many had nowhere to go so they loitered around the city. Temptation was everywhere. They tended to linger too long in the local fast-food restaurants.

Sam left the shelter, and found his way half way across the city to a place to eat, a doughnut shop. He sat there with three other friends at one of the tables near the large window. They looked out at passersby and commented on them as they walked. Everyone seemed to enjoy people watching while they were drinking their coffee or eating doughnuts. That one was too tall, that one was too short. Oh, that coat did not look right. Oh, that one must be homeless too. Hey, he has cigarettes, let's go ask him for some. Oh, there is Norman who owes me two dollars from months ago. He said he would pay me back when he got his paycheck. Well, he must have gotten many checks since then. Let's go ask him for my money. Oh, that one just got out of lock-up. They should have kept that one in there longer. Yes, we all enjoyed people watching and commentary, no matter our circumstances.

Esther drove to the doughnut shop to see Sam. It was easier for her to drive here than to drive across the city. It seemed that nowadays, with all the road constructions and detours, getting to the shelter was not a straight route any more. By the time she detoured and turned and turned, she could not figure out how to get to where she was going.

Esther, our mother, was used to finding and meeting Sam in all sorts of places. If she could drive there she would. If not, she asked her brother to take her there. Russell, her brother was good at that. He was always willing to take Esther when she asked. She figured he loved driving as he had driven trucks and trailers all over the east coast of the United States. During the time when Sam was in a psychiatric hospital, Russell was a lifesaver. The hospital was too far for Esther to drive. The shortest traveling distance in time and route was by the highway. It made sense to take the highway there. However, Esther never drove on the highway. In fact, she had never even tried to go on the highway. There were too many cars and too many lanes. She could not tell if she was coming or going—North or South, East or West. None of the highway signs made any sense to her.

Russell willingly took her at least once a week, if not more often, to see Sam in the psychiatric hospital. This was one of many psychiatric hospitalizations for him. But this time it seemed that it took longer for his mind to come back right.

"His head took him!" Esther would say when anyone asked where Sam was. "His head took him!" No one quite knew what that meant. They thought that there was a problem with his head. Over time, they figured that Sam must have had a "nervous breakdown," whatever that meant. It was not specific enough for anyone to figure out what exactly was the problem.

To Esther this was all "doctor-speak" and it meant nothing to her anyway. Yes, she understood what was meant by sadness, depression, anxiety, panic, hearing voices, and seeing people that were not necessarily there. But, psychosis, delusions, paranoia, hallucinations, bipolar, schizophrenia, catatonia, what was that? What did it all mean? Why did Sam have this condition anyway, what caused it? She swore it was the marijuana that caused it all. If Sam had not taken that first puff and it must have been a bad batch.

Years before Esther had walked into Sam's bedroom and asked, "What is that smell?"

"Sam, is that weed, is that marijuana?"

"Is that ganja, is that "sensi," whatever you all call it?" she asked.

"Don't tell me you are smoking weed?" Esther repeated. Sam was seated on the bed and his eyes were a glazed red. He did not answer.

"Yes, I am sure that is weed."

She walked over to the drawers to go through them. If Sam had marijuana, she was sure she would find it. She flung socks, tee-shirts, and underwear wildly out of the drawers.

"Don't tell me you have weed in my house and that you are smoking it," she said. She wildly flung shorts and short-sleeved shirts out of the drawers to the floor. She was frenzied. If marijuana was anywhere in there she would be sure to find it.

"Don't tell me you are smoking, not weed, not weed?"

She was too intent on her task and she forgot to lift the paper lining in the bottom of the drawers. Finally, something clicked. She reached under the lining to see what was under there. Sure enough, there was a wad of marijuana in a small plastic bag. Esther grabbed it, put it in her pockets and then stormed out of the room. Sam did not flinch as he was so stoned. He was floating in another place. The same could not be said about Esther. She was angry and she went to the bathroom to dump the weed in the toilet. She smiled when the small dark seeds and distinctive leaves were flushed away.

"Oh, Sam, why marijuana, why weed? Don't you have enough problems already?" she asked herself.

Therefore, when she went to visit Sam at the psychiatric hospital and the doors closed behind her, she wondered about the role of marijuana in his condition. What would she do if Russell did not bring her weekly? These weekly trips also were not completely necessary. Sam's mind was so foggy that most of the time she could not follow his train of thought. She would start talking about one thing and he would answer and go off on a tangent about another.

"Don't tell them I am suicidal," Sam said.

"If you tell them I am suicidal, they will keep me here longer."

"Well, are you suicidal? If you are feeling that way, why won't you tell them when the doctors and nurses ask? Did you tell the doctors that you are feeling that way?"

"No, I tell them no," Sam said.

"Why?"

"Because they will keep me here longer."

"Well, you have been here for six months already, and I think you are in the best place right now. At least the doctors can treat you here. You don't have to be homeless on the streets. And you don't have to deal with the police because of you wreaking havoc on everything and then being charged with breach of peace, or worse."

"The police are the ones' who should be charged with breach of peace. They are the ones' who breached the peace!"

"Well, okay, let's forget about that for now." She should have known not to go down that path with him, as the most likely outcome would be his becoming agitated and saying how the police had wronged him.

"So, what did you do today? Did you go to group? Did you have an art class or music therapy? What did you do today?" Esther asked in order to change the subject.

"Oh, nothing."

"Did you shower? Did they tell you to take a shower and change your clothes today? Because it looks like you need to take a shower and change your clothes. Did you shower?" she asked again, raising her eyebrows.

"Oh, yes, I showered and changed my clothes," Sam said. Well maybe in his own reality he had showered and changed his clothes. In this state it was not unusual for him to be completely unaware of his body odor. Everyone else could tell that Sam needed to take a shower. He was oblivious to that need.

Esther knew that Sam had not showered for days. Sam was starting to smell very ripe. It was the same smell that an apple gave when it first started to rot. It was a musty sweet apple rot smell. Sam had not showered and had not changed his clothing for days. Esther estimated that it must have been at least two days of that. If only the workers would just toss water on him and force him to bathe. That was never allowed and she was sure that was not part of any good therapy. Esther also guessed that Sam would not cooperate. She figured that he had not gone to any of the therapy sessions that the hospital offered. Sam was probably having thoughts of suicide. But, if he did, she was certain that he would not tell the doctors that. He might even be hearing voices or seeing things or people that were not present. However, Sam had grown accustomed to all the questions and the reasons why he would not get out of the hospital. He knew that if he said he had thoughts of suicide the doctors would keep him longer in the hospital. Sam would therefore deny the presence of any such thought if anyone asked.

The doctors, nurses, and staff knew that. It was not what you only said. It was also what you did not say. They observed behaviors and the body movements to get the whole picture. Part of the evaluation of Sam's mental progress was the return of coherence in his thoughts. Did he participate in activities? Was he more social or only wanted to stay in bed all day or in his room? Was he paying better attention to his hygiene? Did he take a shower and change his clothing? If he refused to shower, change clothes, and looked disheveled, one could make some reasonable assumptions about his mental state. If you were completely unaware of your body odor, what else could be going on in your mind?

After this prolonged hospitalization, Sam was homeless. Going to the homeless shelter was good, but Esther only hoped that he did not have to leave so early in the morning to wander the city, or to sit in the doughnut shop all day.

Esther parked the car in the lot. Not many other cars were there. She sighed and slammed the car door shut. Was it the marijuana? Was it something else? What made him have these mental problems? Could she have done something differently? She fingered the dollars in the palm of her hands for an answer. She made sure the money she brought for Sam was all single dollar bills. The total amount was only ten dollars. Sam had always told her the money had to be in small bills, and that loose change was preferred. It was easier and better to pay with the exact change. And don't let his friends see that you gave him money or how much, she remembered. Otherwise, that potentially was another source of problem for him.

What was it that caused him to be a person affected by schizophrenia? Some of the doctors said schizoaffective, and others said bipolar disorder? Is that what the doctors said? What was it? Was it the marijuana? Was it me? Was it something that I did? Was it me? Esther really wanted to know.

Empty Nest

Mrs. Simon was still saying that she was in pain. Nothing we had done seemed to make a difference. She was still on patient controlled anesthesia, PCA, and using the epidural spinal catheter that we had placed in the operating room. The nurses in the Intensive Care Unit had called me to rewrite the PCA orders. We had already increased the basal rate dose in the epidural several times. The basal rate was the background rate at which the pain medication was dripping into the spinal canal to control her pain. I had increased the bolus dose that she could self-administer and give herself with the PCA. I had also changed the frequency, how often she could give herself the dose. But, nothing helped. *Nada. Rien.* Nothing.

I looked at her belly first and it did not seem swollen. My stethoscope was hanging off my shoulder, and I pulled it off then tried to warm the bell by gently rubbing it on the sheets. I listened with my stethoscope over her belly. She had active bowel sounds that were not muffled or high pitched. I then placed a gloved hand on her belly to press to see if there was pain on doing that. My hands were always cold and I did not want Mrs. Simon to leap off the bed because of me touching her with freezing hands. There was no change in her expression when I did any of that.

I wanted to make sure that Mrs. Simon did not have another bowel obstruction. I also asked the nurse and an aide to help me turn her over. I needed to look at her back. I needed to see the epidural catheter. Was it still in place or had the catheter moved out of its location? If that had happened, the medication would not work to control the pain, and that may be the reason that nothing seemed to have helped.

I removed the bandage covering the place on her back. The skin site was clean and there was no redness, pus or signs of infection. The catheter was still in place and coming between the bony prominences on her back. Those were the bones that you could feel when you ran your hand down the middle of your back. I looked at the colored markings on the catheter that showed how much of the catheter was inside the space, and marked how much should be out. The catheters had standard markings along its length so that once it was in place, you could determine if the catheter was dislodged because the marking at the patient's back changed. It was still at the same mark and length inside the canal and that part exposed to the outside world.

I didn't think that was it. The medication should be working, but nothing helped her pain. Everyone has a different pain tolerance. Some people could stand a lot of pain and others none at all. It was an individual experience and no two persons were alike, except of course, identical twins. But even then, they may experience pain differently.

I was somewhere in the middle. Some people would say that they could deal with the devil breathing fire down their backs and not flinch even an inch. They could hold their own, be stoic, and not be moved. They could tolerate pain and adversity and come out unscathed. At least that's what they said, that they had no scars.

I wondered about the football player, or any athlete, who still played with injuries and should be in obvious pain. They could charge and sack and attack and take pain and inflict pain while on the football field. They obviously had a high pain tolerance. Yet, in the emergency room, when we were trying to place an IV, or a nurse was giving an injection, the football player would pass out at the mere sight of a needle. They would swoon and do a dying swan. The nurses, doctors, and staff would look at each other and think, "You must be kidding me, right?" One man's strength was another's Achilles' heel.

But, not all pain was the same pain. Giving pain and taking pain were not the same. Physical pain and emotional pain were also not the same. And just because you could tolerate adversity in one setting was no guarantee that you could tolerate adversity in another. If you want to know about pain, then ask me. Right now, I was in emotional pain. What was I going to do? Mom had called me last night at midnight.

"Sam is on the streets again," she said.

"He is homeless and living on the streets. I don't know what to do," she said.

"Well, how did that happen?" I asked. Well, that was a dumb question, I thought to myself. How does homelessness ever happen? Even if I understood the events that led up to him being on the streets, how would that change the plan of action now?

Well, I need to get him off the streets, I thought. But how could I do that? I was three thousand miles away and still at work. I could not simply just jump on a plane the next minute and be on the East coast. I was not superman and I was not Scottie. I could not be beamed up and be there in a jiffy. It always seemed to work in Star Trek. But this was real life. I couldn't really leave him on the streets, could I? All the other relatives and friends had somewhere to stay. Could I do that and live with myself?

First, I was not even sure that the diagnosis was correct. In school they first said that he had a behavior problem. Then it was that he had a drinking problem. Then it was that he had a diagnosis of schizophrenia, then bipolar disorder, then schizoaffective disorder. Oh, he had a dual diagnosis, remember? That meant that he had a mental illness, as well as an alcohol or substance abuse problem. Yeah, I got that. But which one was it? How could you treat the condition if the diagnosis was not even correct?

Dr. Eva Peters was also on call tonight. She was working in the Surgical Intensive Care Unit, one floor downstairs. I knew that Eva also had a brother who was a psychiatrist in Chicago. He was involved in research and had an interest in schizophrenia. In passing she mentioned that her brother treated persons in whom the diagnosis of schizophrenia was uncertain.

I asked her if her brother took on patients that did not live in Chicago. I told her that I had a friend with schizophrenia and that the diagnosis was in question. I grew curious as she told me about her brother being involved in schizophrenia research. If I only could send Sam for an evaluation with him but, how could I do that? First, he had public insurance. If a similar, less costly, equivalent evaluation could be obtained in the state he resided, most likely it would not be approved for payment in another state with an out-of-state provider. I could not afford to pay out-of-pocket for a second opinion. I decided that I would tell Eva that the "friend with schizophrenia who needed help" was actually my brother. I had never done that before as I felt that if I told anyone I would be betraying his right to privacy.

Who talks about mental illness anyway? Who revealed that they have a mental health problem? This was one of the last frontiers in medicine. I struggled with the disclosure myself. If I told my friends and colleagues that I had a sibling, a brother, with mental illness, then would they raise their eyebrows at me too? If there is a genetic link, would they also think that I am at risk? Would they start to treat me differently?

What about disclosure to my insurance company and at my work? What would the insurance company do with that information? Once in their database, would it eventually be used against me or him? But, if we do not start to have this open discussion, how does one overcome the stigma of mental illness?

I decided to go out on a limb.

"Eva, I know you are busy in the Surgical ICU, just as I am up here in the Medical ICU. But can I bend your ear for a minute?" I asked.

"Sure," Eva said. "Do you want to come down here to talk? I can't leave the floor right now."

"I can't either. This will be fast and I will get to the bottom line, STAT."

"Great."

"Look, the friend I said had schizophrenia is not a friend. It is my brother," I said.

"Oh?"

"Yes. And look, he is now homeless and living on the streets. I think I should leave at the end of June and go back home to help."

"Oh? How is that going to help?"

"Well, I can't leave him on the streets."

"Well, if he has schizophrenia as you said, that's a chronic condition. He is not going to get better any time soon. He needs to take his medications. Why don't you get him to Chicago and see if my brother can see him?"

"Yeah, I thought about that too. But I cannot pay for his treatment without insurance. I cannot pay out-of-pocket. I don't think your brother would accept this case and not get paid. I would think he would want payment. Plus, even if he would do this pro bono at first, eventually I would need to pay him. I would feel obligated to pay him for the evaluation."

"Well, Gary, I do not know if that is the right decision. I mean to leave now. You are stopping your work and career to fix something that will be very hard to fix. Schizophrenia, if that's what he has, is a chronic condition. But, I know every obstacle in life is there for a reason. Try to figure out how to overcome it."

"Yes. Let me see if I can figure it out."

"Gary, people make life sacrifices all the time in life and in work. Women do that all the time with family and older parents. Women are used to that and, in fact, are expected to do that. I think that it will all work out. Do what you think is best and it will work out."

"Teach me the power of sacrifice, that's what my mother always said," Eva added.

"You will figure it out, Gary, you will figure it out."

"I've got to get back to work and to the patients," Eva said. "Call me if you need to talk more."

"Teach me the power of sacrifice," Eva softly said as she quietly hung up the phone.

TIP BOX 2

1. Fill your bowl with the large stones first: family, good friends, education, work. Then you can fit in the smaller ones

2. Get plenty of good sleep and physical activity. It will help you face challenging days ahead

3. Intuition: If you sense that something is wrong, it probably is. However, get the facts and information to support your intuition

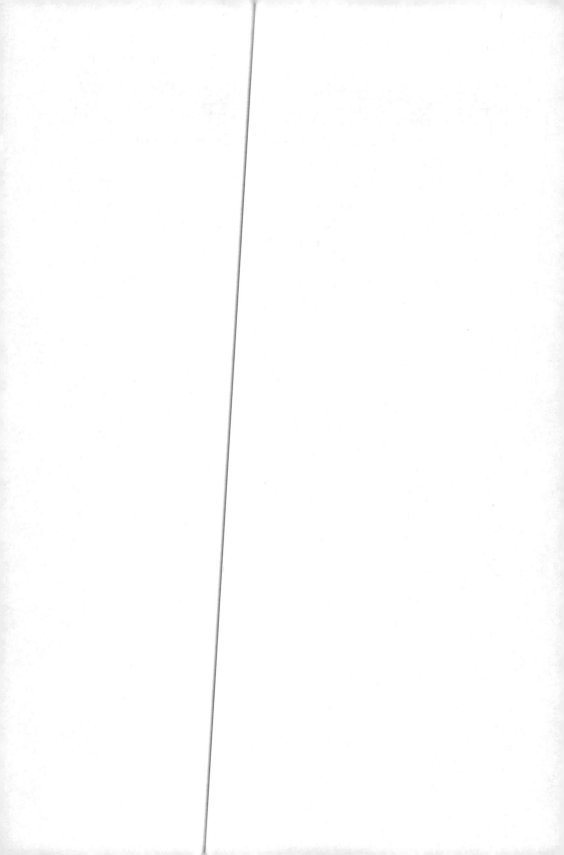

PART III

———————

STORM CLOUDS

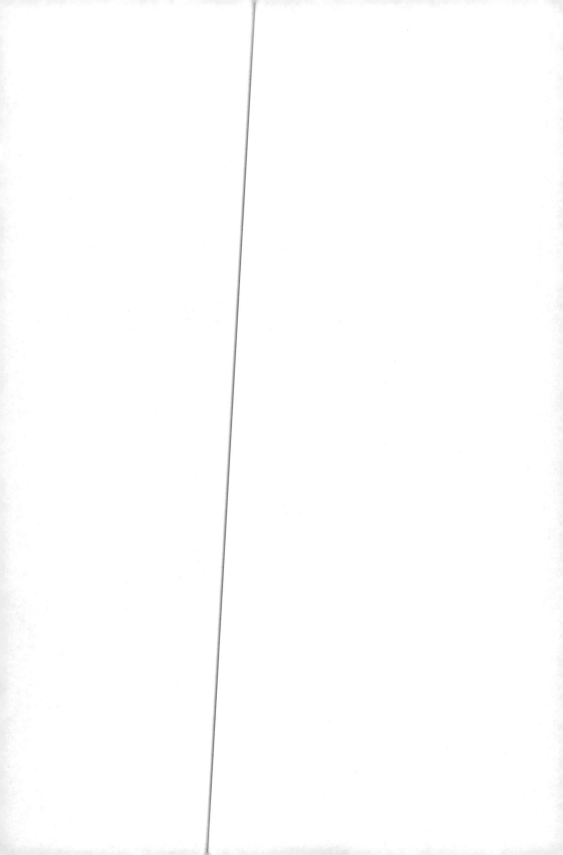

Lunaception

I twist my hair above the horizon

Spiked antennae to the moon

Interference from passing cars as I connect with the universe

Who knows you?

Zoom…

Kneel in the grass to tilt my head

Passersby stare to see if I'll make this here knoll my bed

Mind control the wheels to give me room

Once upon a time I rode a magic broom

All pain disappear when I feel the gloom

Thoughts unravel as they crisscross time

I carry bags to trap the grime

All sweat and dirt accumulate

They know my story and can relate

Catch me now…

Why even stop to ask me why

Connect my thoughts will circuit break

My story is not that I am filled with hate

I have no guns or knives on me

My mind is gone

My family knew

I am homeless you see

And lost my way…

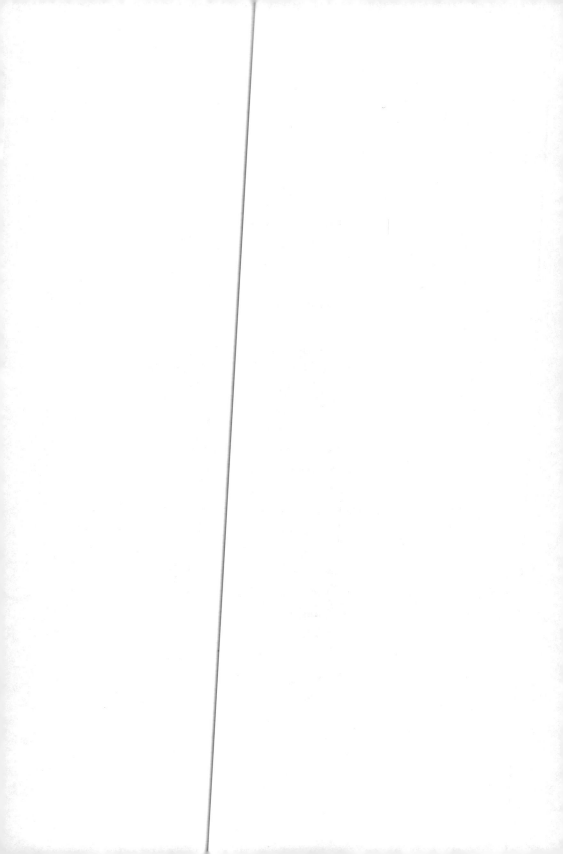

CHAPTER 9

EARTH AND SKY

I attempted to get to the telephone before the fourth ring. I did not want the answering machine to pick up before I got to it, as it was programmed to answer after the fourth ring. This was an older phone and there was no caller ID that announced the caller's name and number. If it did, I could choose to ignore the call if I did not want to talk to anyone at all. Luckily, I did not have that problem often. I was very circumspect to whom I gave my phone number. I had also opted out of telemarketers' databases. I did not want to have some random marketer calling me at nine o'clock at night about a product or a service that I did not want. Luckily, I grabbed the phone on the third ring.

"Hello," I said.

"Hi, it's me," she said dejectedly. It was Esther.

"Sam is in jail again."

"Okay? So what happened this time?"

"Well, he was at the club. I think he must have been drinking. He loves that beer. You know I tried to stop him from drinking. I keep telling him that his brain can't take alcohol. Plus, it knocks out your liver. He always gets "out-of-whack" when he drinks. You know, those who can't hear, will feel. Having "hard ears" is not good. If you won't listen to your parents' good advice, your fingers will get burned more times than they really should. You know what I am saying?"

"Okay?" I responded. I waited for her to make her point. I had heard this lecture many times before. It stuck in my brain from all the times that I was warned about not listening to good advice. How it was not good not to listen to and take feedback, whether the feedback was good or bad. With aging comes experience and knowledge. Yeah, ask somebody who has been there. Take a walk in their shoes and you will know that what I am saying is true. They can tell you what it is like to live that life.

"So why is Sam in jail this time?" I asked. I was trying to bring her back to why she had called in the first place.

"Well, he was drinking."

"Yes, Esther, Mom, you said that before." I wanted her to get to the story.

"Why is he in jail this time, Mom?" I repeated.

"Well, it is just more of the usual. He was drunk at the club. Mr. Jacquin said that he started to cause a ruckus. He was screaming at the top of his voice. He was getting into people's faces, standing too close to them, and invading their space. Mr. Jacquin, of course, knows him, tried to get Sam to go outside. Well, he would not listen to Mr. Jacquin. You know how Sam can be stubborn. It's like you are talking to a stone wall. He started talking about how the world was coming to an end and he was getting people nervous. He said that the end was near. You know. He was talking fast and talking too loudly. None of it made any sense," she said.

Okay, I thought. Being loud and annoying should not land you in jail. We have all seen the man on the street corner with a bull horn yelling: "the end is near, the end is near, repent, repent, repent!" That did not land the man in jail. It did not even mean that that person had a mental illness. Rarely, would the police pull that person off the street. I don't even think people think of it as a breach of peace. Sam probably had also looked dirty. I imagined his hair was not combed and that it was matted. He probably was unshaven and had a body odor from not bathing and wearing the same dirty clothes for weeks. I imagined what he looked like. A loud talking rambling man telling you that the end was near. It was not something that was endearing. In fact, it was downright scary. Most people would become extremely uncomfortable around that.

"Well, something else must have happened," I said. "For them to lock him up, I mean."

"They said it was for breaching of peace."

Sam was arrested for breach of peace because he would not listen to Mr. Jacquin. He became belligerent and talked loudly. He was still talking loudly when the police arrived. When they got there Mr. Jacquin tried to tell them that Sam had a "problem."

The police officers who came knew Sam well. The last time these same officers had arrested him because he threw a brick and broke a car window. He had not been drunk then. At that time Sam was hearing voices and he said that "someone" told him to throw the brick into the windshield. He had stopped taking his medications. He did not take them because he said that he did not like the way the medications made him feel. I assumed that the medications ordered his thoughts and stabilized his mood. When he took the medications the noise and the voices in his head were quiet. There would be no voices forcing his actions. That must have been an unusual experience to have his thoughts ordered. Maybe he did not like that. He had grown used to the voices and the chaos in his head. Some people thrive on chaos and disorder. If things are ordered they feel like a fish out of water. The chaos was like an old welcoming friend.

"Oh, we know Sam well," one of the police officers said. This had been the third time that month that the police had been called. Sam had been involved in some activity where he was annoying someone, disturbing the peace, or breaking things. It was a never-ending cycle.

"We will take care of it," the officer said.

"The end is near, the end is near," Sam said to the police. He willingly put out his hands to have the cuffs placed on them. The officers obliged and did not argue with him as Sam was not always this cooperative.

"The end is near, the end is near. Yes, officer, please arrest me. I have done bad things. The world is coming to an end because of me," Sam said.

"I have done bad things. People have no work because of me. It's entirely my fault. I've done bad things. The end is near, the end is near," Sam said again. The police officer quietly led him away and placed him in the back of the police cruiser.

Sam would want to voluntarily take the hit for bad things happening in the world and in people's lives. The economy. Unhappy friends. Joblessness. Angry people. Homelessness. Depressed relatives. You name it. All the bad things he would assign to himself. He thought he was the cause even when you told him there was no link to him. None whatsoever. I would try to reason with him that none of that had to do with him. He did not control the economy. He did not control whether people had jobs or not. It was not even because of one man or one thing. Sam did not create the universe or the earth or the sky. None of this had anything to do with him. You can surely change the world. But first try to control your little corner of it first I would tell him. None of that made any sense to him. He felt that it was because of him the world was coming to an end.

"So, he is in jail because he was drunk and caused a breach of peace," I said to Esther.

"Yes," Esther said, "and the cops are sure tired of seeing him. So he is in jail now. I am sure when he goes to court tomorrow the judge will "throw the book" at him."

Esther was right. When the judge saw that he was here again in front of him, he sentenced him to one year in the correctional institution. In retrospect, I think that was a good thing and a bad thing. At least there he would get the psychiatric care that he needed. He was in a locked place in prison and the nurses would make sure that he took all his medications. His thoughts should become ordered with the medications. But, in prison what were the costs? The prison system was probably not the right place for him. What he needed was to be in a locked psychiatric ward.

I wasn't asking for the earth and the sky. Was that too much to want? Was that so unreasonable to ask? To ask for an appropriate place and care for his mental illness that was not in prison?

Engineered for Failure

When Sam was released from prison after a nine month stay he had no place to go. He could not go to live with Esther as she was living in a one bedroom apartment. In the past she allowed him to stay with her when he called to say "can I stay with you for a minute?" He would live in the living room. Soon, the "minute" turned into hours and the hours into days. The days turned into weeks. The apartment was too small. He would become agitated and he could not sleep. He would stay up at night pacing the floors. When she was trying to sleep he came into her room telling her that he could not sleep. He would have to go soon. Otherwise, the other tenants and the management company would start to complain about an additional person in that small space. Sam did not melt into the background as he was conspicuous because of his appearance and his behaviors.

"Mom, are you sleeping? I cannot sleep," Sam said.

He would do that like clockwork every ten minutes. Of course, she could not sleep. First it was from the constant interruption. Then it was from him coming into the bedroom and standing over her bed. It was not that she was afraid that he would harm her. He had never been violent towards her or threatened her before in any way. But she wasn't naïve. She slept with her car keys under her pillows. She was not going to let him get anywhere near the driver's seat of her car.

She knew that she had to be vigilant at all times. Even the most docile of pets, cats or dogs, have been known to turn on their masters and loved ones without notice. Sometimes it was without the slightest of provocation. Maybe it was a change in your scent, hairstyle or clothing. Something that was subtly changed about you that was unrecognized by you. But they had a preternatural instinct that you could not identify and that you could not recognize. They too were hyper-vigilant and hyper-aware. They could easily sense your fear, your disdain, and your naiveté.

Then there was always the "breaking news" on television. The newscaster would describe the story about the son, or rarely the daughter, who killed his parent. Who knew what was going on in Sam's mind? There could be some unknown trigger that not even she was aware. What was it that might cause him to "lose it"? But, she was determined not to toe dance on eggshells in her own home. She did not want to become a prisoner in her own mind and life. She refused to be locked up and immobilized from fear and shame. But, Sam paced all night and she would get no sleep. In the morning she would be completely exhausted and irritable. Before the work day even started she would be cranky and angry from the lack of sleep. She avoided her co-workers merely to prevent taking any of that out on them.

Despite not being afraid of him, and sometimes allowing him to stay with her, she knew that for now, it would be better for Sam to go to the homeless shelter. He had been to the homeless shelter before. She thought that would make more sense. Besides, what would he do alone in the apartment when she went to work? Would she come home to find pots burned on the stove? He was forgetful. He may put on a pot or a kettle on the stove and forget that it was there. He needed to be monitored and she usually did not allow him to use the stove at all. What had happened since he was in prison? She did not allow him to do some things alone at home. Would he remember not to turn the stove on? What did they do to him in prison? Did he take his medications from the doctors and nurses without a fuss? If he committed a crime she felt that he should be punished. However, she thought that being locked in a prison cell was not always a good thing. She knew he needed constant psychiatric care. He was much better when he took the pills. Did they provide that kind of care in the prison? What did they actually do for him in there?

She was also older now as well. What she could do when she was thirty years old was not what she could do at fifty. She was not as physically able to do all the activities that he needed help with. She could still try to protect him from himself. That was a mother's instinct to serve and protect. That was also the police's motto, to serve and to protect. Is that what they had done for Sam in prison? He served time because he was drunk in a public place. He was breaching the peace. He became loud and boisterous due to the drunkenness. The judge looked at how many times Sam appeared before him. Sam had become a public nuisance. Something had to be done. The police and judge were serving and protecting the wider community and public. But on an individual level, who was going to serve and protect someone who obviously needed psychiatric care. What was the root cause of the drunkenness? Sam had an underlying mental illness. If that was not addressed, no amount of prison time would fix that. Did the police and judge even see and understand that? Was he referred to psychiatric care? How did you get to the root of the problem to fix it if you did not even know what it was?

The shelter was happy to have Sam back there as he had been there before. This shelter only accepted men. Homeless women and families were referred to one that accepted families. But like many shelters in the city they were overburdened and overworked. Often, there were no available beds. Some of the men and women who sought shelter there were not from the city. People complained about the "prison bus" that would drop off in the center of the city those who had served their times. Some of them had never even been to this city before. They had no family here and no social ties to the city. But word-of-mouth was a familiar way to get the word out to those who needed to know. The homeless found themselves at one shelter or another. They relied on the kindness of strangers, and they cherished the friendships they had formed while prisoners together. Like it or not, it was an informal society that few of us will understand unless we are in it.

The homeless transitional program gave Sam a single room. As far as shelters go, this one was fairly well organized. He had a case manager assigned to him. The shelter also had created partnerships with local health care agencies. They had health care providers that would come into the shelter to provide nursing care and give medications. There was also a medical provider to see the clients who needed onsite medical care at the shelter.

However, with most shelters, you had to leave after breakfast at seven o'clock in the morning. You were not allowed to come back in until six in the evening. The only exceptions were if you had a medical excuse that allowed you to stay inside. These were few and far between. That's not to say that many clients did not try to get a medical excuse. That way they would not have to leave the shelter during the day. The providers would see many clients who would want the health care provider to write the medical exception letter. The claims would be that they could not walk, could not move, needed a softer mattress or needed to be given two meals rather than one. And the list went on and on. The rookie health care provider would write the first two letters. Then the pattern would become obvious. It was the same people every day and every week who needed an excuse. He would catch on to the game very quickly. He had to become astute at figuring out who really had a medical need and who really only needed motivation. Malingerers were everywhere. Sometimes he got "played." But, if he stuck around long enough to learn the ropes he would know what "once bitted, twice shy" meant.

Being put out in cold or rain or in the middle of winter motivated many people to become actors. They would create elaborate scenarios to increase their chances to get a medical excuse. Exaggeration and hyperbole were useful when you were "playing the dozens" with friends. It did not work too well with the doctors, physician assistants, nurse practitioners and nurses. It worked even less so with the shelter's staff. They had seen it all and heard it all before. The stories usually did not work with them. The staff could tell who needed an excuse even when the client did not ask for one.

"Are you kidding me?" Sam asked. "You mean I have to leave now and come back at six?"

"No, I am not kidding you," Barnes answered. "And yes, you have to leave the building. You know the rules. Out by seven, in by six. At least you don't have to stand and wait in line for a bed. You are in the transition program. Your room is assigned."

"But, I don't feel good," Sam complained.

"Where am I supposed to go? You gotta be kidding me. What about my meds? What about my meds? When will the nurse come?" Sam asked. Barnes stared blankly at Sam and chose his words carefully to respond to Sam.

"The nurse will be here soon. Once she gives you your morning meds, you will be all set until this evening. You can walk and talk. Your body is good. Lying in bed all day is not good for you anyway. You can take a walk to the park and hang out with your buddies there. We don't have a work assignment for you yet. When we get you on a work assignment then you will have some place to go. For now, you will have to go hang out with your buddies. Go to the park and see what's happening there. Take a sweater as it might get a bit cool. You will be all right. You know the drill. You have been through this before," Barnes said.

"You gotta be kidding me. Where am I going to go?" Sam asked again.

Sam asked the same questions for the next five minutes. Barnes patiently gave Sam the same responses. Eventually it would sink in. Barnes had also been through this before with Sam. Reinforcement of information was a good thing. Barnes was calm. Rather than becoming angry, upset or frustrated, he gave him the same answer. Eventually it would sink in. It had to. Once he got tired of complaining Sam would walk outside. He would go with his friends to the park or roam the streets until it was time to come back into the homeless shelter at six.

The Rent Is Due

Lola stood over Sam while she took his blood pressure. She took it twice to convince herself that the reading was correct. It was really as high as what she had gotten when she took it over the sleeves of his shirt. Huh. She was definitely right the first time.

"Sam, are you taking all of your medicines?" she asked.

"Yes," he replied. "I take them."

"Do you take all of them?" she asked again.

"Yes. Vanessa comes every day and gives them to me."

"Who is Vanessa?" Lola asked.

"She is the visiting nurse. She comes and put them in the pill box."

"She or Gary waits until I swallow them before she leaves," he added.

Vanessa, the visiting nurse, did in fact come every day. She poured the medications and watched Sam to make sure that he had swallowed the pills. She would stand there and made sure that Sam had not cheeked the meds. I did the same thing in the mornings. Sam had done that before, pushing the pills there to hide them under his cheeks. When she was gone he would spit them out. He would do that when he thought that no one was looking. Vanessa knew that it was really important that Sam take his anti-psychotic medications. If he did not take these medications in short order you would notice a change in his behavior. First, he would start to become withdrawn and depressed. Then he would start to talk less and less. Eventually, he would start to hear voices, hallucinate and become delusional. He then would start to talk more. But none of what he would be saying would make sense. His mental state had been good for the last six months. So Vanessa wanted to triple check to make sure that Sam was not hiding the pills in his mouth.

"Open your mouth," Vanessa insisted.

"Are you sure you swallowed them?" Vanessa asked. "Lift up your tongue so that I can see." Vanessa had gotten on well with Sam. He did not give her a hard time. He got along with this nurse as that was not always the case. He wanted to fire several of them that came. You could not predict who he got along with and who he did not. One of them he disliked on meeting her for the first time. I don't even think she had said more than a few words. He would refuse to take the meds from her. He must have sensed something about her. But what? Another he fired and I asked him why. "I didn't like her eyes," he said.

I did not condone that behavior as he felt he could hire and fire them at whim. In my book he did not have much of a choice. But, if it came down to fighting with him to take the pills, the battle was not worth it. There had to be a compromise. Win the battle to lose the war? It was not worth it. But, he liked Vanessa and he did as she asked. It had made our lives a whole lot easier. Lola, like Vanessa, paid attention to the small details. And today, Sam's blood pressure was really high.

"Well, let's go to see Heather now," Lola said.

Heather was Sam's clinician. She was the licensed clinical social worker who treated Sam and she was the lead in his therapeutic sessions. She worked with the psychiatrist, Dr. Aldrin, who saw Sam monthly. Aldrin prescribed Sam's medications that kept Sam's mind clear. Lola walked with Sam to Heather's office and handed her the paper work with the blood pressure circled in red. She wanted Heather to notice that it was high. Heather looked at the numbers and did not say anything. She decided that she would let Sam rest for a while and then she would ask one of the nurses to take the blood pressure again.

"Sam, please sit and give me a second," Heather said, and got up to speak to Lola.

"What are you doing about your own blood pressure?" Heather asked. "Lola, did you go to the clinic to have your blood pressure checked again?"

"No, not yet."

"Well, why not?"

"I have been too busy."

"How do you mean?"

"You know I work all the time."

"Well, I know. But I told you that the community health center has late hours. They are open up to 7 p.m. in the evening. They are even open on Saturdays."

"I know."

"Your blood pressure was really high that last time."

"You need to get that treated. We don't work on Saturdays. Why don't you go then?"

"I will," Lola lied.

"Okay, go this Saturday to get it checked," Heather urged.

"Yes, I will, I will go this Saturday."

Lola did not tell Heather that she would not go at all. Lola felt that was the least of her problems. Lola was worried about getting all the money to pay her rent this month. She was only working part time now and the job did not provide her with insurance. When she went to the doctor she had to pay out of her own pocket. She did not have the money to go to the clinic to get her blood pressure checked either. She knew that she needed to be on medications to get her blood pressure down. Heather had told her that the community health center was not going to charge her a lot. Heather even told her about the sliding fee scale. She could pay based on her income, if she had to pay anything at all.

"What am I waiting for? Why am I stalling?"

"I have a family history of high blood pressure. I always figured that my time would come when I needed to take pills to get this under control. I know that I use too much salt in my food," Lola talked to herself. "I know that I need to increase my physical activity. The last doctor I went to told me to take the blood pressure pill every day. She even printed out and gave me the DASH diet, Dietary Approaches to Stop Hypertension. I know what to do. I know that I must do this for me. Why am I stalling?" Lola asked herself again.

Well, for one thing, she was taking care of her elderly mother at home, and she was doing that by herself, Lola thought quietly. And for two, this part-time job did not provide medical insurance. Besides, and for three, the rent was due. She was living with many stressors and it was as if she was swimming upstream against a tidal wave. She was swimming, but not moving, and getting absolutely nowhere. It was as if she were a lifeless plank in the water.

Lola's mother was in the early stages of Alzheimer's. "All-timers," as she called it to herself when no one was listening. She had taken her mother to her doctor and the doctor had confirmed it. It was a good thing that her mother had Medicare, the health insurance for the elderly. She remembered Medi-CARE for the elderly and Medic-AID for those who needed help because of their income. It was a good thing her mother had Medicare to pay for the tests. The doctor ordered a CAT scan of the head before he felt fairly comfortable saying that her mother had Alzheimer's disease.

CARE for the elderly and AID the needy. This was the only way Lola remembered which insurance was which. She was a health care worker, but the two constantly confused her. CARE for the elderly, AID the needy. When she did it that way it was easy to remember. But taking care of her mother was not easy. When Lola was alone, she felt frightened, ashamed, and anxious. When she went to work she left her mother home alone. "It is no wonder my blood pressure is through the roof," she thought. "I have all that stress, and I don't feel like I can tell anyone about what is going on in my life. My rent being due is really the least of my problems," Lola thought.

Lola first thought she noticed a problem when she went with her mother, Angela, to vote. Her mother, who had voted all of her adult life, did not know what to do with the ballot. Lola told her mother to darken the circles in black ink for the candidate that she wanted to vote for. When Lola looked at the ballot, her mother circled the entire candidate's name and did not darken the circles.

"No, Mom. I said to fill in the circles. Not to circle the names," Lola said.

"No you did not," her mother insisted. "You told me to circle them."

"What? I did?" Lola asked.

"Yes you did, you did!" Angela said.

"Huh," Lola thought. "I must have given her the wrong instructions." But Lola started to notice other things as well. She noticed that her mother, Angela, started to have lapses in memory. Lola thought, "Well, that's not news. I also sometimes cannot remember where I put my house keys or if I paid a bill or not." But then it became more obvious when her mother seemed to forget the simple things. Her mother would get up to go to the kitchen to get an item. Or she would put the kettle on the stove and forgot that she was the one who put it there. It happened one time too many and Lola knew something was not right.

Her life was not *"Like Water for Chocolate."* She did not think that she could withstand the obligation to remain single to take care of elderly parents. But, sometimes what you don't want is what you get. It was the law of attraction at work. If you feared a thing so much that it consumed your mind, you attracted it to yourself. Free your mind and enjoy your life. That's what her mother always told her.

Lola had no other siblings. She was it. There was no older sister that Lola had to stand in line behind and wait for her to get married first. Lola luckily would not have to watch her older sister marry some man that Lola loved. She did not have to cook any meals for her sister and her husband. She did not have to wither away and stand by silently suffering looking at her sister and her spouse. Lola had no boyfriend and she had no other life to speak of either. Angela's life. That was it. That was also Lola's life. But, at least she was spared the burden of unrequited love.

Lola was the only child and it was only her and her mother. Lola's father was completely out of the picture. But, that did not just happen yesterday. That had been the case for most of her life. Lola did not speak to her father. She did not even think that if the chance came that she even wanted to talk to him. She was certain that her father was here in this same city and state where she lived. She did not seek her father out and he did not seek her out either. Lola thought that she could easily find her father if she really wanted to. But she was certain that she did not want to. "Stalling for any reasons? No."

Lola was not stalling. She only felt that she had no time to take care of herself. The doctor told Lola that in the early stages of Alzheimer's the person has problems with thinking and remembering. The person could also have problems with reasoning and problems completing daily tasks like dressing, bathing, and eating. Lola had already taken over paying her mother's bills and handling all of her accounts. But, while Lola was at work, she would worry about coming home to find her mother lost, wondering the streets and not being able to find her way back home. Lola hoped that if that happened when she was at work, her neighbors would show her mother back to the house, or allow her to sit with them until she came home. Lola was always watchful and always on the edge. She had her guard up at all times and she observed everything about her mother. Lola walked through every room when she got home. She had to see if anything was out of place. If something had changed, Lola wanted to know early. Surprises. She could not cope with those. Surprises? No.

But who was Lola fooling? Could she even think she could do this alone and still go to work? Her mother's doctor was very good in providing information and explaining that it is a good idea to seek out family and support groups. Well, there was no family to seek out. She was it. He told her about Alzheimer's disease, its progression, and the need to start planning. The doctor had told Lola that the memory loss and confusion may get worse. Her mother may start to have problems recognizing family and friends. Lola had to work and take care of her mother. When would she find the time to go to a support group?

How could she do that when she felt that she could not tell her neighbors or co-workers what was going on? Why should she even tell them? She was not asking to be treated differently. She knew her job and did it well. If she started to tell them this information they may feel she is looking for an excuse. This was far from the case. She just needed someone else to talk with and to share her experience. She knew she was not unique and did not want special treatment. She pulled her weight and always had. But many hands made work lighter. If she had some help at home it would be such a big help.

Lola's mother was not in the late stages Alzheimer's where she may start to see mood and personality changes. She was not in a stage where her emotions could suddenly change and at the drop of a hat uncontrollable tears would start. She was not angry and argumentative all the time. Lola was grateful for that. She had to already cope with co-workers who brought their issues of depression and control into the workplace. Some were always angry or depressed and found negativity in everything. Others you could not give feedback before they would start crying what she thought were useless and unnecessary tears.

She promised herself to save her tears for situations where it really mattered, when she would grieve for a friend or a love one. Others were simply manipulative, did not pull their weight and never looked inward to see how their own actions affected you. They had no self-reflection and no empathy. They probably were very narcissistic as well. She was grateful that her mother did not have these personality issues. She coped with enough of that at work. She walked on eggshells at work not to offend anyone or start problems. She could not also do the same at home.

Her mother's doctor told her to start planning for the future. He told her that in the severe and later stages of Alzheimer's her mother may not be able to communicate. Her mother would then be completely dependent on her and others for her care. Lola made up her mind that if that happened then the only option she saw at that point was to put her mother in a nursing home. She was anguished over that thought. For her mother to have a life it meant that she may end up not having one. Was that her only option? Lola did not ever remember her mother pointedly telling her that she loved her unconditionally, or that she was thankful for all that she did. Now that her mother was "losing it" she was doubtful that she would ever hear those words spoken out loud to her. But some things you simply knew and felt deep down inside and speaking the words were not necessary.

"Well, I know, Tag, I'm it. I am just not ready to cope with it now though. I'll cross that bridge when I get to it," Lola said. "But God, please help me when I get there."

CHAPTER 10

YOU WILL NEVER KNOW

Jodie slammed his right fist hard into Sam's jaw. His aim was perfect as he made connection with the angle of the jaw. The bony prominences of the cheeks and the jaws cracked, and yielded to the force without any protest. All the power crashing into Sam's jaw was also transmitted to the left side. The left side also creaked and snapped as it was unable to absorb the full pulsating energy from the assault. Jodie then pounded the left side of Sam's head with the beer bottle that he held in his left hand. The beer bottle shattered as it contacted the solid casing of Sam's skull. Shards of glass from the beer bottle fell unceremoniously to the ground. A spring of bright red blood squirted and pumped from the broken blood vessels on Sam's head. The blood jumped for joy, happy to be free from its place of confinement.

"I told you to give me your cigarettes," Jodie said. "Next time, give me what I asked for. Give me the cigarettes."

Sam was on his knees, writhing in pain, and could not respond. His jaw was loose and freely floating in his mouth. If he had tried to speak now it would only be mumbled and jumbled words that came out. The blood sprang from somewhere on Sam's head, and more blood gushed out of his mouth.

"Next time give me the cigarettes. Or give me some money. I know you just got your check and money from the state," Jodie said. Sam clutched his jaw, and he clamped his left palm over the place on his head from where he thought the bleeding came. These actions did not make a difference. The bleeding would not stop coming from either place.

"Hey, stop, stop it, Jodie! Stop it! Why did you have to hit him?" Conrad asked.

"Stop it, man! Look, now he is bleeding!" The other men who were looking on wanted to yell out the same thing. But Jodie was a bully. He was bigger in body, more muscular, and had spent more time in prison than the rest of them. He was always angry and the simplest of things would set him off. He walked around scowling. Conrad knew that Jodie had an anger management problem. Hey, they were all prone to speaking loudly and getting upset at something or another. Jodie, on the other hand, just seemed to take his anger to the extreme.

"Hey! Stop, we have to get him to the hospital. Look at what you just did?" Conrad said.

Fortunately, the hospital was only a few blocks away. The men were hanging out on the streets in front of the community center, and across from a doughnut shop. This was the cozy spot where all the men hung out until it was time to go back to the homeless shelter. In warmer weather they stood outside under the trees and "shot the breeze." When it was cold, they sat in the center, or in the doughnut shop. They tried not to disturb the patrons, especially in the winter; otherwise, the workers there kicked them out to stand outside in the cold and snow.

Gemma dashed across the street and dodged oncoming cars. She had to see what was happening. She had been peering through her office window and had seen the quick one-two jab. However, she had not seen the bottle that Jodie had delivered to Sam's jaw and head. Gemma was the social worker on duty today at the center. For the next twenty-four hours she was on-call for the "mobile crisis" hotline. She knew that she had to constantly watch the men and see what they were up to. This was especially true on the first of the month as there would always be fights. The fights were because the men would have gotten money from their disability or social security checks. Sometimes mothers, fathers or siblings would come by and also give the men money. That money was meant to last for thirty days. On the first of the month it was debt pay-up time. It was also a good time to bum a cigarette or two.

Some of the men were in a constant state of begging and borrowing. It did not matter what time of the month it was. They would spend all the money in a day or two. What was there to save for? Some of the men were caught in a perpetual cycle from the streets to the prisons. Why even think about the future? When their minds were clear and more lucid, they could not even imagine looking ahead to the next day. When their minds were unraveled, they could have experienced and lived in the present, past and future all in one day. They only knew today and they lived in it. They learned what to do to survive and they had to quickly learn survival skills. In the streets they had to learn to survive or they would die. The men could cajole and manipulate to get you to give them what money or cigarettes or food that you had. Some were experts at that. Some were less skilled and willing to accept help. Many of them would allow the social workers to manage their money for them and help them to pay for rent, for food or for other supplies. But some of the men were paranoid, fearful or untrusting. Others were always angry and aggressive. Some, like Jodie, were menacing. If you refused to yield to their demands you could be subjected to an unexpected physical assault. The best advice was to not stay around that type. Unless, you were skilled at de-escalating conflict, your best bet was to run. Run—don't walk—when you saw the likes of that menacing kind coming. Sam had often said that if he saw Jodie first, he would duck and hide. He would go in the other direction, any direction. This time though, Sam was caught off guard. Today he had not seen Jodie coming in his direction. By the time he saw him it was much too late.

Despite what we believe that everyone with mental illness is frequently violent, the opposite is true. Persons with schizophrenia and severe mental illness were more likely to be victims of physical assaults and injury at a much higher rate than the general population. But, of course, they could be the perpetrators as well. Some of the injuries are self-inflicted, especially when they are in a psychotic state. They could harm themselves or harm others.

Persons with schizophrenia or other severe mental illness often sought refuge in emergency rooms for many reasons. It was a place that they could come to for help, to calm the mind and soothe the body. Even when they resisted the help, the medications and help they could get there, were not always available in the community. Because they also were at higher risk of being victims of assault, the emergency room was a place of solace from others who would inflict injury and assault them.

"Oh, no," Gemma said. She was careful not to address or to talk to Jodie directly. She surmised that Jodie had been off his meds. But, even when he is on his meds, he was angry, belligerent, and argumentative. She continued to ignore Jodie and flipped open her cell phone.

"We need an ambulance," she said. "Yes, across from the doughnut shop. Yes, it's a man. He was hit in the face and the head. Oh, it looks like it was with a beer bottle. Yes. He is breathing. He is bleeding from his head and mouth. Yeah, he is awake and sitting up. Oh, I don't think he can talk," she said in response to questions the dispatcher must have been asking.

"Five minutes?" Gemma asked. "The ambulance will be here in five minutes. Okay." Gemma stood there watching the men and she thought that there was nothing more that she could do at that point. She had no gloves or bandages and nothing to press on the wounds. There was nothing immediately around her that could stop all that bleeding. "Five minutes," she said again, trying to calm herself down.

By the time the ambulance arrived, Jodie, like snakes are prone to do, had slunk away unnoticed. The ambulance attendant was very good at placing an IV. He found a large vein in the crease of the arm, and with one fluid motion placed an 18-gauge needle into the vein. He pushed forward the small plastic catheter, or tube, that would remain to keep the vein open. He secured the plastic catheter with tape, covered it with a large bandage, and hung a small bag of saline to keep the vein open. With such a large intravenous, the attendant was sure the vein, with the steady flow of salty water, would remain open. The size of the IV turned out to be a good choice to give pain medications, fluids, antibiotics and blood products, if needed.

Sam was bleeding from every orifice on his face, except from his eyes and ears. He was obviously bleeding from his mouth and his nose. At first, it was just the gush of blood, and then it became a steady stream. Now, the bleeding had slowed. However, it did not seem that the bleeding was sufficient that a blood transfusion may be needed.

The attendant radioed into emergency services control to ask for pain medications. He described the situation and the injury. When the doctor came on the radio, the attendant recited the vital signs, the blood pressure, and heart rate, and he said, "This man had a severe blow to his jaw. It is probably broken. I am calling for permission to give something for pain." The doctor on C-Med control approved the request and the attendant said, "Great, see you within five minutes, Doc."

Coming into the emergency department by ambulance this time was a charm. Sam was lying on the stretcher, and he sat forward as this made it easier to breathe. It also made it so that he would not swallow all the blood and could spit it out into the pink plastic basin the paramedics had given him. It was more like drooling the blood into the basin as he had no control of his jaws. He could not really spit. The bony jaws would not move in concert assisted by the facial muscles for him to have control over the spitting function. He could not really speak either. Everything was mumbled and jumbled. His jaw was freely floating and freely mobile.

By the time Gemma got in touch with me, told me what happened and where Sam was headed, the ambulance had already picked up Sam and taken him to the emergency room. I arrived shortly after Sam was placed in the room, and just before the nurse and the ambulance attendant started their exchange. Scott K. was the nurse assigned to this room. You could not make out the last name on his name badge as he had put tape to block out the last letters of his name. Scott came in to the room to take the report from the ambulance crew. The first paramedic handed Scott the written report that stated the time on scene, the problem, the vital signs and what treatment the ambulance crew had initiated. Though the attendant was speaking, Scott was obviously only half listening. He was reading the written report and seemed not to have any interest in a verbal report. Apparently, the paramedic did not notice Scott's lack of interest in a verbal report and therefore, he kept on talking.

When the paramedic finished speaking, Scott hardly looked up or looked at him. He placed the report on a small counter and went to the right side of the bed. He inspected the IV site. He flicked and turned the small plastic bag to see what type of fluid was hanging, and he opened a drawer that was below the counter and pulled out three glass tubes. There was one red top, one blue top, and one purple top, and he busied himself to get blood from the IV site.

During all this activity, Scott was expressionless showing no emotion. His demeanor was flat and his motions were robotic. No muscles in his face moved. Neither his eyebrows nor lips twitched. Now satisfied that his initial tasks were completed, he labeled the vials and placed them in his pocket. I don't remember him asking if Sam needed more pain medications. Scott turned on his heels and it was obvious he was about to leave the room. "Are you in pain?" Scott never even stopped to ask the question. Scott pivoted on his heels, turned, and left the room, slightly slamming the door on his way out.

"Schizophrenics just need to get their act together!" Scott muttered much too loudly. Of course, my ears were already peaked and ever vigilant for signs of danger. I had to hear him.

"Was it as simple as that?" I asked myself. "Schizophrenics just need to get their act together?"

I glanced at my watch and realized that I was going to miss my scheduled appointment with my own doctor.

On the heels of Scott leaving, Dr. Keney walked in. He was too tall and too lanky. He looked like he was a vegetarian and must be a runner. Unlike some people who avoided meat and insisted that they always ate healthfully, he did not look that healthy. In fact, he was too thin and his gaunt appearance made him look older than how old I thought he was. I assumed that his appearance probably had to do with his living with chronic stress. This was only my assumption. For some reason or another, we had never gotten to the point where we were that comfortable to talk about our own lives outside of work.

"Oh, Dr. Gary, it's you," Dr. Keney said when he entered the room. "Of course, when I saw the last name, I thought the patient was you who was assaulted and injured. I did not pay too much attention to the first name of the patient in the room," he said.

"Well, maybe next time you should!" I muttered under my breath. Unlike Scott, he had his name badge with his full name spelled out. His badge read, Dr. Rene Keney, MD, Emergency Medicine. The combination of his two names was odd. I did not think that he was French, nor did I think he was Irish. I don't even think he spoke a lick of any foreign language, or for that matter that he had ever left this city. He never spoke about any vacations that he took or going anywhere to visit family or friends. Then again, as I said, we did not have that kind of friendship, if you can call it that. It was more colleagueship. But, now in retrospect, I had never heard him say that he was away from the city visiting anyone, anywhere, anytime.

Despite his gaunt face that conveyed severe unhappiness, he was extremely pleasant. He stretched out his hand to greet me and to say hello. His hands revealed that he was an academic. There were no callouses in the palms and the hand muscles were not well developed. If he was used to hard work it must have been through mental exercise only. And he must be used to working very hard as his face and demeanor showed it. Whatever made him stressed and gaunt looking did not involve him having to use his hands repeatedly to do any labor. His fingernails were kept very short, were clean and neat. There wasn't a speck of dirt under his fingernails. Though his palms were not calloused, the skin of his hands was dry and scaly. The scaling was due to his constant washing and use of the foam antiseptic. He didn't take much time to moisturize them with lotion after work as the scaling seemed like this was from days of lack of lotion. Maybe he was too busy at home to do so, or he just did not care about the appearance of his hands. The same could be said about his face. He did not seem to want to have to do with anything that took too much time. He wore a military crew cut and his blond hair was starting to turn gray. The hair at his crown and temples stood straight out looking like bamboo reeds that were stiffen, inflexible, and unyielding by age and time.

"Hey, Dr. Gary, it's good to see you. You got lucky today, huh? It is hectic in the emergency room today. There are patients everywhere and they just seem to be coming out of the woodwork. They are hanging from the rafters. Everybody is sick or injured or something. I just can't seem to keep up today. Thank God my shift is almost over."

"Oh, hey, Dr. Keney, good to see you too."

"Oh, I thought it was you, Dr. Gary, who was injured," Dr. Keney said again.

"No, it's Sam. No, it's not me. See. It's my brother who is injured," I added. "Look. His jaw is broken."

"See, Dr. Keney, I can talk. Sam's jaw is broken and both of the handles of his mouth are freely floating. He is drooling and there is blood coming out of his mouth. Sam can't speak. See, Dr. Keney, I am speaking and talking to you," I said to myself without speaking it out aloud.

"No, it's Sam," I said. "No, it is Sam that is injured. See his jaw is broken. Dr. Keney, you are obviously busy. Let's page the oral and maxillofacial surgeons, OMFS, that is. They can finish examining him. They can order the CAT scan of his head, face, mandibles, neck, and jaw to assess the extent of the injuries. Obviously, he needs to be admitted. Once OMFS knows the extent of the injuries they can take him to the operating room, repair the jaw and whatever, and wire the mouth shut."

"Dr. Keney, you know with this type of injury, it is a slam-dunk admission. Let OMFS complete the work-up, and they will admit him. You also know that his jaw will be wired shut for six weeks," I said.

"Dr. Keney, you look harried and you are clearly tired from what looks like the shift straight from hell. Call OMFS and they will take care of it," I repeated. "You can move on to your next patient, and maybe you can complete your work, and get out of here on time for a change."

"It is a nice day out there, get out of here on time for once," I said.

"All right, all right, I hear you."

"You are right. I will have Scott page OMFS. That way the oral and maxillofacial surgeons can finish up and I can get out of here early," Dr. Keney said.

"Yes. You do that. You got an easy one this time."

"Page OMFS and have them wrap things up for you," I said. Sam's jaw will be wired for six weeks. To have my jaw wired for six weeks and having to drink only liquids out of a straw was not my idea of fun.

"Yes, you got lucky," I said. Now confident that the admission would go smoothly once OMFS was on board, I glanced down at my watch.

"Look at the time," I said. Time just seemed to have run away from us.

"I am going to miss my appointment again with the doctor. Oh, well, next time," I said to the air. "Yes, I got this too," I added, to give myself comfort that it would be okay to miss that doctor's appointment for the second time.

Speechless

Sam's jaw was wired shut for six weeks as the broken jaw needed time to properly heal. Jodie was not a professional boxer. Yet, the blows that Jodie had delivered to Sam's jaw had transmitted a furious destruction that was only equaled by Jodie's perpetual high of unmanageable anger.

Sam was forced to take only liquid foods and drink through a straw for the duration. The oral and maxillofacial surgeons had given me wire cutters, and they were only to be used in an emergency. They said that if needed in an emergency, for example, if Sam was choking, or we needed access to his open mouth, or if he were not breathing, then I had to use the wire cutters to open up his mouth. Of course that meant that after that was done, Sam would then have to have the wires replaced. I hoped that there would not be any such emergency. Drinking through a straw was not such a big deal, right? Some people may even secretly want to be able to drink through a straw. The rationale was that they would lose some weight during that period of time. The only thing about having your mouth wired for six weeks was that it left you speechless.

But, Sam was used to being speechless, so to speak.

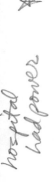

I thought about the time that I had sat across the administrative judge in a large and cold conference room to complete the conservatorship papers. About a month before the hearing I had received the notice in the mail. The hearing was to discuss whether Sam was competent to take care of his affairs as he was about to leave the psychiatric hospital. The claim was that he was an incapable person, not capable of making his own decisions about his health or his finances. There was no way that the doctors and health care providers would allow Sam to leave the hospital after being there for almost a year and a half without the conservatorship being done. He was to be discharged to a homeless program that also operated a respite program.

The state sent petitions to the interested parties to be present at the hearing. I went with Esther. The court-appointed lawyer was there but the psychiatrist did not show up. He probably did not need to. He submitted all the clinical information about the diagnosis, the long history of mental illness, repeated hospitalizations, treatments, and prognosis, in a thick document to the court. However, Sam' clinical social worker was there. She was always there for Sam—no matter what. Rain or shine. Mountain top or valley low. Heather was there to support Sam and to help us decide on what the best course of action would be.

Judge Shelly Wallingford started the hearing. She spoke in a high soprano voice and she gave a pleasant but curt greeting to all present. You could tell that she was the no-nonsense, take no prisoners type. I interpreted her calm, professional demeanor, as the "don't-waste-my-time" type. I certainly had no intention of wasting the judge's time. I was also very busy. The sooner we got this over with, the better we all would be. Judge Wallingford flicked her finger and punched a button to start a small tape recorder.

"Oh," she explained, "We record these sessions to make it easier for the court clerks to transcribe and record the events. That's the only reason for recording today." The court appointed lawyer and Heather nodded. They were already aware of the process. Esther and I also calmly nodded in agreement. Did we really have a choice? We were players on the judge's chessboard. It was Judge Wallingford's court, her turf, her game. She exuded I take "no nonsense and no crap." She made the rules. She called the shots. She moved the pawns. We would have to play by her rules.

"Yes," she continued. "We are here in the matter of Sam. This hearing is for the application of conservatorship of the person and estate." She looked around the room at each of us and said, "For the record, each of you, please clearly state your name and title or relationship to Sam." We identified ourselves. Judge Wallingford inconspicuously laid the tape recorder on a pile of papers that was on the desk, and the machine recorded quietly. You did not hear the slow whizzing and winding of the tape around its spool. We all tried to speak clearly and loudly so that our words were not muffled.

Judge Wallingford seemed to be looking over the documents and reams of paper that the psychiatrist from the hospital completed. She already read and knew the diagnosis: Schizophrenia, chronic, recurrent, mixed type, Bipolar Disorder II, Alcohol Dependency, in remission. The global assessment of functioning in the last year was twenty percent. This was the GAF score and it was very low. Dr. Terry, the psychiatrist probably also had written that Sam had a long history of mental illness with multiple hospitalizations. He

memory

probably wrote that Sam had poor judgment, poor insight, and poor memory and was forgetful of recent events. However, Sam could recall in vivid details events from the past. Most of these events that were in immediate recall were traumatic. There were other times when Sam had problems with impulse control. He needed supervision in all his activities of daily living, like bathing and preparing meals. He needed to be supervised in the kitchen, for example using the stove. The psychiatrist's documentation went on endlessly for pages and pages. Judge Wallingford glanced up from the page and stared directly at us. It was obvious that she had already read over the details of the case. She looked at the papers again to jog her memory.

Everyone at the table was quiet and waiting for her to guide us in the discussion. It was amazing that when you knew that you were being recorded that you attempted to order your thoughts. You also made every effort to enunciate and speak clearly. At least you had to try. The discussion etiquette was excellent. We tried not to interrupt and cut each other off when someone else was speaking. Then again, Judge Wallingford ran a very tight ship. You really only spoke after she addressed you directly. Maybe all communications in life would be improved if they were being recorded by someone, somewhere.

"Doctor Gary," Judge Wallingford began, "Attorney Bernard is here because he is appointed by the court. You stated that you are willing to be appointed the conservator of person. That means you would make the decisions about all his life activities except his finances. That is, you would be directly involved in all decisions about his housing, health care, and the like."

"However, in matters of his finances, money, bills, and the like, you could let Mr. Bernard be appointed to do that, if you wanted. If you choose to also have control over his finances that means to be appointed conservator of estate as well"

"Do you understand what that means?" the judge asked.

I nodded. "Yes, Judge, I know what it all means."

"It means that you would be responsible for handling any money or funds he receives, and administer those money to pay his bills, buy clothing, food, personal care items and other items that are necessary. You would also need to submit periodic reports to the court about how that money was spent. Are you willing and able to do that?" the judge asked.

"I am sure you received in the mail the summary booklet on conservatorship sent to you by the court and what it means. I assume you read the booklet and know what it means?" she asked.

"Yes, Judge, I have read it and know what it means."

"Therefore, are you willing to be both conservator of person and estate for Sam?"

"Yes, I am."

"Sam, are you in agreement to give conservatorship of person and estate to Dr. Gary, your brother?" Judge Wallingford asked Sam directly. Sam nodded yes. He did not speak.

"Do you have any questions about this, Sam?" the judge asked him again.

"No," Sam responded this time.

"Is there any further discussion on the matter?" the judge asked.

Everyone at the table leaned forward to look at the judge. Those quietly swerving in short and narrow rotations in the swivel chairs, or leaning back and forth on them, stopped to pay attention. But, we said "no" together. "Okay. Therefore, we will appoint Dr. Gary as the conservator of person and estate for Sam."

"In the next couple of weeks, Dr. Gary, you will receive a court document with the seal affixed that you will keep as evidence of this hearing. You should also provide copies when needed to health care professionals and others involved in his care that may need this document. Okay. So, if there are no further questions, and no further discussion, the hearing is now closed. Thank you for coming. It was nice meeting all of you. Please have a good afternoon," Judge Wallingford said.

Therefore, when Jodie broke Sam's jaw leaving his mouth wired for six weeks, as well as speechless, I walked around with wire cutters to open his mouth in order that he could speak, or breathe, if needed in an emergency. Where were your wire cutters? Who among you willingly wants to be conserved in person and estate? No one intentionally wants to be speechless. Or do they? To have someone else make decisions for you. How will you know if your best interests are being considered? Were you even consulted before the decision is being made on your behalf?

The Jodies of this world may deliver that sledgehammer blow when you least expect it, and when you are most vulnerable. That would leave you without a voice, speechless, and without someone else to stand up to speak up for you. If you choose to be speechless, six weeks is much too long a time to intentionally allow it to happen. How about if it were a lifetime? No one ever chooses to be speechless, and I yearned for the day when the likelihood of that occurring diminished.

CHAPTER 11

A PIECE OF COOKIE

I t was more than perfect. All the stars were in perfect alignment this morning.

I got out of the emergency room at the end of my shift on time, for once. It was still very early in the morning and I was very much awake despite not sleeping for almost twenty hours straight. I tried not to make a habit of going that long without sleep. However, my sleep deficit would continue for a couple more hours. I was looking forward to a long day where I could get multiple things done before my next bedtime rolled around. It was very early in the morning, exactly 6:30 a.m. I was already walking in the skywalk that connected the hospital building and the third floor of the parking garage. I was skipping with delight happy to get out of the hospital at that hour. It was not uncommon to be there one to two hours after the completion of a shift to complete the paperwork and the charting in the patients' medical records.

At other times, it was that a conversation with a patient or family member became complicated and had taken winding turns. You wanted to answer all their questions and let the patient know what was going on. Or sometimes, you waited to talk to another doctor that you had paged to tell them about their patient that you had to admit, or discharge and needed follow-up, or for another specialist's input. The return calls or conversations did not happen on a schedule as you would have liked. They did not know that your shift was done at six o'clock and that you were ready to go home.

It made sense for you to stay and to talk to the patient or doctor. There was no point in you giving that information to the doctor that was relieving you as they were not involved in the case in the first place. By the time you gave the summary to the relief doctor, and they reviewed the information, something was lost in translation.

You made a risk versus benefit assessment. It was practical to clean up after yourself, complete what you started, and then hand off a completely finished product. No one likes to clean up your unfinished work. Unless, of course, you are at a natural gap in the process. At that point anyone could easily take over. Yes, they smiled and said it was okay. But, even when they smiled and said they would do it, you could still hear the muttering of disgust under their breath. You agonized over wanting to leave on time, but when you took pride in your work, you did not want to leave unfinished work. It was similar to the mason, who much like an artist, liked to complete the stone work that he planned, designed, and created. He did not want to leave it to someone else to complete.

I was happy to get out on time, this time. I worked the overnight shift from 10 p.m. the night before to 6 a.m. this morning. Dr. Setelar, the doctor for the shift starting at six o'clock arrived on time, and he was scheduled to work until 2 p.m. We all preferred these eight-hour shifts. The twelve hour ones were hit or miss. If it got busy, as invariably it would, by the eleventh hour, you were running on fumes. All the petrol and gas in you were completely drained.

Yes, Dr. Setelar was on time. He was extremely punctual and came early every day. In fact, when I looked up from the computer at 5 a.m., and saw him, my heart jumped and raced with joy. It was early, and my replacement was walking into the department.

I wanted to yell out, "Will someone please hire him. He is the best worker! Ever!"

Now, reaching the end of the skywalk, I opened the door to the parking garage, and walked onto the third floor. I always parked in the same spot as this was one thing fewer to remember. If I did not park on the third floor, I went to the fourth and parked in the same place. I did not want to arrive in the parking garage, fumbling with my keys, and then spending the next five minutes wondering where I parked. From that point, I would waste the next ten minutes walking from floor to floor looking for my car. No. No. No. Time was of the essence and I had none of it to lose today.

I was already suffering from a sleep deficit. Those fifteen minutes lost and wasted meant fifteen minutes less of sleep, of leisure time, or for something else. I walked past a couple of early bird workers who swiped their badges to get into the building and into the hospital. We all nodded "Good morning" to each other without speaking. I guess it was too early to speak and everyone was trying to conserve energy and speech. I found my car. Of course, it was in the same spot. There it was exactly where I had left it. I jumped in the car and did not wait for the engine to warm up.

In less than a minute, I was out of the parking garage and onto the street. I ruminated over the cases and the patients from last night. There was the patient with the heart attack, one with pain from sickle cell, two with migraine headaches, three people with pneumonias, and one kid with appendicitis. I lost track of how many motor vehicle crashes had come in. They all had different types of injuries with different broken bones. Then there was the young woman with the intentional drug overdose. On top of that, there were a couple of persons drunk or high on some kind of substance. There were a couple of broken bones: an ankle, an arm, and two broken hips after a slip and fall at home. There was the man with prostate cancer, and a kid with a small part of a toy stuck in his ear. Then there was another person with a foreign body stuck in a private body part. I did not even bother to ask how it got there. I removed it with long forceps and bid him adieu. That had been my night and I was exhausted.

Oh, there was the man with belly pains. After all the blood work testing and CAT scans were completed, and the results reviewed, I discharged him home. I conferred with his doctor and decided that it was okay for him to go home. Yet, I kept on wondering if that was the correct decision. Sometimes, we doctors ruminated, and ran the case over and over in our heads, and agonized, and wondered if we made the best decision. Was that the right choice? Was there something that we did not ask the patient or interpreted incorrectly? Should we err on the side of caution? Could we live with that decision or would we come to regret it? But, you had to act, gather the facts, interpret them, and make a decision. You could not become immobile by fear and indecision. You had to make a decision.

Still contemplating the night's events while driving in the car, I turned left off one street and onto another. I drove past a homeless shelter. No one was outside on the streets at this time of the morning. The shelter had a soup kitchen. They housed the homeless, and fed anyone else who needed a warm meal. I had never volunteered at a soup kitchen. Esther had done that many times before. Many of my friends had gone to volunteer and to help serve food there. Most of them did that only during the holidays, at Thanksgiving or at Christmas.

But, Albany was different. He was a constant volunteer. Every Saturday, he had gone to the soup kitchen to do his part. Why Albany's parents chose to name him that was a mystery to me. Some people thought it was a travesty of justice, and downright criminal to do that to a child. A name sticks with you for life. If the name was so outrageous, you were compelled to change it, or simply use an initial.

But, Albany was a strong name. It made me think of something that was permanent or a powerful place. I thought it was an unusual name for a person. When asked, "What's your name?" and the response was "Albany" most people would probably do a double take and raise both eyebrows in disbelief. They probably were thinking and saying quietly to themselves, "Who would do that?"

Albany served food to the men and women who for one reason or another found themselves without a home. Sam had been homeless but he had not stayed at this particular shelter. He had been at practically all of the other ones in the city.

However, the homeless shelter in Philadelphia was one of the best I had ever seen. How they had found my number and was motivated to call me was still a mystery. They must have gotten Sam to give them my name and they did some research to find me. With the ever present concern of patient privacy and security of information, everything must remain private. Unless, of course, the patient opts for disclosure. The privacy concerns around mental health and substance use were even more stringent than if it were solely a medical or physical problem. Without the written consent to release mental health information, sometimes parents and families were left completely clueless to what may be going on with their family member.

Sam was notorious for wandering off at the oddest of times. This time he left the city and bought a bus ticket to get out of there. He was going nowhere in particular, but he ended up in Philadelphia. He knew no one there, and by the time he got there he had no money. Luckily, Sam avoided being arrested by the police. He was not arrested for vagrancy, for a breach of peace or some other public nuisance, this time.

At the homeless shelter, he had to sign in at 6 p.m., and sign out of the building at 6 a.m. He was not used to that kind of structure, but he really needed it. Structure, support, and consistency helped to focus his mind, to stay on track, to take his medications as prescribed, and to remain in therapy.

Structure

Just when I turned off the highway exit to Market Street in Philadelphia, Pennsylvania, I turned on the radio. I played only CDs on the drive down to Philly. Now, I wanted to hear the news and find out what was going on locally. I did not find a radio station immediately. There was only an irritating static emanating from the radio and I could bear the grainy noise for only a brief moment. I decided to go back to listen to CDs and what I was certain was music that I liked. The music that I brought along for the ride soothed my mind, and prevented my thoughts from racing and thinking about what I might find at the end of this trip. I listened to the music for the positive messages, inspiration, and upbeat tempo.

I put the same CDs back in the slot and listened to the same songs for what probably was the tenth time on this trip. The up-tempo beat of the songs lifted my spirits. I silently tapped out the beats on the steering wheel in syncopation. Doing so steadied my heartbeat. Ah, the sound of the music. It was soothing and calming. The songs gave me a sense of peace and calm that I sorely needed after the long drive down from Connecticut. What kind of shape would I find Sam in at the shelter? Would he recognize me? Would I recognize him? Would he have his hair cut and his beard shaved? Or would I find him dirty, grimy, and unkempt?

At some fleeting point of mental clarity Sam must have given the staff at the shelter my telephone number. So mentally, he could not be that bad off. Or did the staff inadvertently find on him the telephone number when they were going through his belongings in order to secure them? Whatever thought or clue brought them to find the telephone number was really fine with me. It was a miracle out of the blue. Some things are gifts and need not be questioned.

I parked on the street a little away from the shelter rather than trying to find a parking lot. I had to walk half a block back to the entrance as there wasn't a free space immediately in front of the entrance. The shelter's door was open. I walked up to the reception desk and told the man why I was there. After I signed in the male clerk behind the desk haphazardly waved and pointed to the elevator where I would go to the second floor to see Sam. I punched the up button and waited. In a minute, the elevator's gray door creaked open. It was the only elevator to go to the second floor. I did not want to spend time looking for the stairwell even though taking the stairs would have been faster.

I entered the elevator and looked at the numbers on the panel of buttons. This elevator must have been put in the seventies. The space was cramped, and only two or three people could fit in it comfortably at any time. If more than three people entered you would be pressed too closely together. Some people get into your space to talk to you. But, in an elevator or any small space like this, it would be creepy, and you would have to overcome the urge to push the other person out of your space. I breathed a sigh of relief, and was thankful that I was the only person in the elevator. I pushed the second floor button to get the elevator going. The elevator's doors noisily creaked shut.

"Okay, okay. At least it's moving. Old doesn't mean that it doesn't work."

When the elevator doors opened on the second floor I breathed with pure joy. I looked around at the second floor to see a wide open space that served as a recreation area. Once off the elevator, I could see that the room was divided into four sections. Immediately in front of you, sofas and chairs were arranged in a circular fashion to appear as a living room. Once seated each person could easily look directly at another. I assumed this was an area for a social gathering or meeting.

In the corner to the right was an enclosed area with a large counter. The counter top was made of black laminate, and it was wide enough to hold glasses, plates, and trays. There was no one at the counter now. Behind the counter and in the partitioned area was a kitchen area that housed a shiny new restaurant grade commercial grill. It had lots of burners and a double oven. A large refrigerator, a sink, and several iceboxes filled out the rest of the space. I walked over to the kitchen attracted by a brightly colored dedication plaque on the wall. It read: "In Memory of Pearl Fordhart. For with love, all things are possible." This space and grill was donated by the Fordhart's family in their mother's memory. I was excited by this act of generosity from this family given so that the homeless persons who used this space and obtained a warm meal could walk in a path of inspiration and love long after the physical person for whom it was donated was long departed from this life. Most of them probably did not know this woman, but she was hopefully able to play a part in their mental health recovery.

As I stood admiring the plaque and the shiny grill, Cathy Earle walked over to greet me. Cathy was the manager of the shelter. She was short, thin, but had a booming voice. I put out an outstretched hand to greet her and she took it and shook it forcefully.

"We are glad you came," she said. "I am the manager here. I was the one who found your number in Sam's shirt pocket. It was on a crumpled piece of paper. It only had "Gary" on it. I decided to call to see if we would reach someone who knew him. I knew that he was not from around here. I used to live in Connecticut, so I knew that the 860 area code was from there. I have been working with the homeless for fifteen years or more. We know most of the men and women who come to seek shelter here. I knew he was a newcomer. I am glad you came and he is doing a lot better. We took him to the emergency room and the doctors gave him some medications," she said.

"How long has he been here?" I asked.

"About two weeks, going on three," she said. "He was in a bad mental state when he came in and we had to take him to the emergency room. After the doctors saw him, they kept him in the hospital for a few days. He was no harm to himself or others, but he had racing thoughts and was actively hearing voices. They gave him medications to stabilize his mental state. The social workers arranged for him to come here after he was stabilized and referred him to the local clinic to continue outpatient care. We had him seen in the outpatient mental health clinic for other therapy and continuing medications."

"We are glad you came," she said again. "Sometimes, when we call families, they do not come. You know, they have lives too. And being involved with and caring for a family member with mental illness is very stressful. Not everyone can cope with it, and not everyone should. It is very stressful. That's why we are here, to help and to support you."

families needed ☆

"A lot of times, by the time the person with mental illness gets here, they have burned all their bridges with families and friends. They may have sold the families personal items, threatened or harmed them, been abusive or simply refused help. But for the person to really recover, and recover well, the person needs support and the families need support. None of them can really do this by themselves and they should not have to." I nodded in agreement. I was glad to come and would be glad to take him home as well.

"Let me go get Sam. He will be glad to see you," she said.

I nodded again and watched as she walked to a door in the far right hand side of the room. The upper half of the door was made with reinforced plastic so that you could see what was happening on the other side. Cathy unlocked the door and walked into what appeared to be the sleeping quarters. I was left alone so now I glanced over the rest of the room. Immediately to my left was the space carved out to be the recreation area. There was a table-tennis table that was folded and pushed up against the wall. A built-in book case housed a small locked cubicle that had the tennis balls and rackets inside.

Across from that area, there were chairs arranged in classroom style all facing a blackboard. For now the blackboard was clean with no writings, teachings, or instructions. There were few if any pictures on the wall. Whatever knick-knacks that were hung seemed to be immobile, secure, and flush with the wall. There were no sharp edges or objects, or loose objects that could be a potential missile. Someone must have gone through the room and thought about every nook and cranny, every fixture, every piece of furniture to create a safer space. The space was multi-use and functional, but the place was designed to create serenity and peace.

Cathy returned with her bubbly smile and effervescent spirit. Sam was walking behind her. His gait was brisk and steady. He was not walking in a jerky staccato manner, so that was a good sign. He was shaved and his hair appeared as if it was recently cut. His face was a bit gaunt and he looked like he had not had a full night of restful sleep yet. His clothes were clean but the pants and shirt were loose on him. I did not think that these were his clothes. Most likely, Cathy and other workers had given him clothes from a donated collection that they kept on hand for those in need.

Sam was moving his mouth around in a slow chewing motion. He was twitching at the mouth and smacking his lips. Sometimes when he was not taking Cogentin with the antipsychotics that cleared his mind, he would appear stiff and twitch. Sam walked evenly towards me and I could see that he was holding a cookie in his hand. He smiled, put his hand out, and offered me some of it.

"Here, have a piece of cookie," Sam said.

I smiled, took the cookie, and held it in my hand. At least his speech was coherent and the words coming out of his mouth made sense. Sam was speaking clearly and offering to share what little worldly possession that he had. That was a good sign. I was glad I came. It would be good to get him back home to Connecticut. Maybe we could hold on to sanity for a longer period this time around.

Looking up the Wrong Tree

Esther sat on the iron wrought garden chair that was on the patio deck at the back of the house. She placed her coffee cup on the round decorative table, and she lightly breathed a sigh of relief. It was good to stop and rest for a quick minute. She loved the chair's new light green color. The last time that Ermelinda was here she had painted the two chairs and the table lime green. Ermelinda was her second cousin on her mother's side. Ermelinda never seemed to stop working. She would work all day long. She would start first inside the house and then she would go outside. When you thought she should be completely exhausted, you would find her outside pruning hedges or planting flowers. She would rake the leaves in the backyard all by herself. Ermelinda never complained about work. Esther tried to tell her to use the blower vacuum, and that would have made it so much easier to gather the leaves. But, Ermelinda was old-school. She knew a way that worked well for her and she stuck to it. She always said "If it is not broke, don't fix it."

Esther had no idea how Ermelinda became a perpetual motion machine. She did not stop working at all. Esther was glad when Ermelinda was around because it took some of the burden off of her taking care of Sam. At least there was an extra pair of hands to do some of the work inside the house.

Esther knew that Ermelinda had a difficult life. However, Esther did not know all the details of what had happened to her. Ermelinda barely wanted to speak about it. But, for one thing, Esther knew that it wasn't until Ermelinda was about thirty years old that she knew that the woman that she called Mother was actually her grandmother. It turned out that Ermelinda's mother gave birth to her when she was only a teenager. No one wanted to talk about why Ermelinda's own mother was not allowed to care for her. Was it because she could not or would not? Or was it that her own mother thought that a young teenager could not take care of a baby. Her mother was really just a baby herself when she had her.

For years even after she knew the truth she still called her real mother Auntie. She could not bring herself to call her "Mother." How could she? Her own mother was practically a stranger to her. Ermelinda did not have the nerve to ask her grandmother why it turned out that way. She assumed that they must have known best. Her grandmother always knew best and did the best she could. She was not ungrateful for the love and care that her grandmother gave but, at some point she wanted to know why. Why had her mother given her up to be raised by her grandmother? Why?

Ermelinda was used to hard work, and there was always lots of work to be done at her grandmother's house. Her grandmother was the go-to person. She always seemed to take in family members, cousins, and friends, you name it. There was always someone in need and in dire straits. Ermelinda knew what it was like to have housing instability or no home at all. It was good to have someplace to turn. Ermelinda knew the value of working and she swore to herself to work so that she never found herself out on the streets. She kept herself busy by doing things inside the house and outside. She reflected on how indirectly living through an experience built a conviction to not let that happen to you. Ermelinda loved to work and she did not wait for her grandmother or anyone else to ask her to do a task. If she saw a need, and a task to be done, it was done, and without complaints.

Therefore, when Ermelinda saw that the small garden chairs and table were crying out for a new coat of paint, she took the extra paint that she found in the garage, and "presto change-o," the deed was done.

Esther looked out at the tree that was in the middle of the backyard. She knew a thing or two about trees and flowers. That type of tree there was strong and it could practically live anywhere. The petals were strong enough to resist damage from insects, and she also knew that these trees needed a lot of care. When the plants were young they needed a lot of watering and care. Without care, water, and nourishment, the trees and petals would not be strong. These petals were beautiful and could withstand damage from all kinds of pestilence.

She knew a lot about cultivation and care. She had taken care of Sam all of his life. When all else failed, she was the one encouraging and cheering and watering and cajoling and healing. What Sam needed was constant and enduring. Sam needed to be nourished daily. He needed help with practically everything; with bathing, grooming, and preparing his meals. She really had no qualms about taking care of him as she had strong maternal instincts. She knew that this was her child. She felt that it was her job to protect and care for him as needed.

However, the constant care that Sam needed limited her social life. In fact, she was convinced that it was one reason why her marriage broke down and ended in divorce. The stress of taking care of a child with a mental illness was too much for her husband to bear. In fact, few of her friends even understood her commitment. Even fewer of them knew of the actual challenges that she faced. There were several times when she was asked to go to a play, a concert, a party. She just could not make it, and she didn't explain a whole lot to them about why she could not go. She just did not go. Most of her friends knew that she had children, including Sam. But few of them knew of the daily tasks and the scope of her responsibilities.

Few of her friends came to her house, and she rarely went to their homes either. There were a few times when she allowed friends to come to her home and into her life. She was not ashamed of her home and she was not ashamed of Sam. She kept her home immaculate and she tried to keep everything in its place. Her house was comfortable and homey. When you live in a state of potential disorder and chaos, you had to try to find a place of order. She had *interesting* ✗

to create order out of none— constancy out of unpredictability and heaven out of a possible hell. Esther wanted to create a place of safety and a place of love. Without that she did not think she could face the outside world. She had decided that if she had to spend so much time at home it might as well be a place that she really could call home.

She looked longingly at the tree. That tree needed a lot of care. She knew that Sam needed a lot of care too. She also recognized that many people blamed her for Sam's mental illness. They didn't have to do that. She had already blamed herself. She felt guilty that it was her fault that he had this problem. Her friends loudly called her an enabler. The health care providers and clinicians probably also did too in their own quiet way. The friends and family all said that if she had practiced tough love Sam would not be this way. Hey. They claimed that they had done tough love with their sons and daughters and that they were all better off for it. Well, were they? Esther was not so sure of that. They accused her of handicapping Sam because she had done too much for him. She was always there to pick up the pieces. But was there another way? She had not seen another way that worked. When she saw homeless men and women on the street, or people with mental illness alone, she wondered about the family. Had they tried and failed? It was overwhelming to care for a person affected by mental illness. If you were doing this all by yourself it could be an unbearable burden. Unless you had walked in her shoes or in similar shoes could you truly understand? Most people didn't understand. Why should they? Everyone has a burden to bear and a story to tell. If you had not experienced what they had, how could you understand? But this was her duty. It was her obligation to care for her child. This was her cross to bear. They say that everyone has one. Until the day that she could not do this anymore she would carry out this work with love and care.

Esther made many sacrifices. She changed her work life. She made sure that when she was out of the house at work that there was someone available to stay with Sam. She relied on the help of family and sometimes a few friends. They had to be comfortable with Sam though. They had to be patient. But they also had to be direct and firm with him. You had to lose that fear that he would be violent. He never was. But many people have the notion that every person with mental illness is violent and waiting for a moment to strike. That was not the case with Sam. But safety was still job number one. Just as you poison-proofed your home when you have a child in the home, you did the same when you had a person with mental illness at home. If you had a toddler in your home, you did not leave household items that are poisons lying around. You did not keep pill bottles everywhere. And you certainly labeled cleaning supplies and kept them locked and out of reach.

Safety was a priority and therefore, Esther rarely had any sharp objects around. You had to be able to think clearly and calmly when under extreme stress. If there were a clear and present danger you had to think quickly on your feet. You could not waver and you could not wobble. Not many people had the right combination of the personality and skills. If you had never worked or lived with someone with Sam's needs it could be overwhelming. It took time and experience not to become fazed by the demands. It did take a special person and they were few and far between. But first and foremost safety was job one.

Esther had given up a lot to take care of Sam and she had done so with minimal help. It was not that she did not need help. At one point after her husband had left, she remembered going into the Department of Social Services. She got the courage to ask for assistance. She sat in front of the social worker who was asking her questions to see if she may be eligible for help. Esther remembered that the woman was very smartly dressed. Her shiny black hair was pulled back into a tight French roll. It accentuated her facial features. Her forehead was high and her eyes were deeply set. Her eyelashes were long and straight. She never blinked. There was an inkling of crows' feet beginning at the corner of the eyes. Her makeup was perfectly applied and her lips were evenly red from the lipstick there. She wore two simple diamond studs in each ear. They sparkled when struck by the light in the room. The collar of her white blouse was crisp and neatly starched and she wore a close fitting pink cardigan that displayed her figure and fit form. There were no wrinkles in her clothing.

The woman looked down at the application that was in front of her. She looked at the type of work that Esther did. She looked at the annual income. She looked at the reasons why the woman was in front of her and in this office today.

"Why are you here today?" the woman asked.

"I wanted to see if I could get some help. I wanted to see if I could get some assistance."

The woman did not reply. She looked up from the piles of paper in the yellow manila folder on her desk. She looked evenly and squarely at Esther. The pools of her eyes were deep and unyielding. Only the red lips moved and the rest of her face was rigid.

"Lady, why don't you get a better job?" she asked.

Esther didn't need to hear anything more. She had heard that one too many times before. Esther pushed herself away from the desk. She got up out of her chair, stood up, pivoted away, and grabbed her jacket off the back of the chair. She walked right out of the doors and felt the woman was spitting darts at the back of her head. She never looked back once. No need to become a pillar of salt. It is always good to know where you stand with people. She didn't stumble and she never faltered. This had been the reaction that she had gotten all of her life. There was never any use crying over spilled milk, was there?

She knew that many people blamed her and they said that it was her fault. Her husband blamed her, and she suspected that her family blamed her as well. They didn't really have to do that. She blamed herself enough. But she knew that with conviction and faith that she would make it. Nothing could break her then and nothing would do so now. She would find a way and create a new path until her very last breath. She would never give up and she would never quit.

She vowed to do all that she could to protect the thing that was given to her. She had a choice. She could make Sam's life a blessing or a curse. She could make her situation the same as well. She knew that with all that she had been through she had learned a lot in her life. She had learned to have patience. She had learned to persevere and to endure. She felt that there were few things in her life that she could not face. Whatever mountains were there she knew that they would be moved. She had faith. But faith without action is nil. She had no fears. Why have fear when you can have faith? She knew what it felt like to feel shipwrecked. But, she was determined to get to land even if it were on broken pieces of the ship. She knew that she had done this work with Sam so many times and through many years. She had become skilled at it. But she was not naïve either. She knew that there would be a point where she could no longer take care of Sam. She worried about what would happen at that point. But, she decided to cross that bridge when she got to it.

"I will prepare for that bridge but I will not cross it before it's time," Esther vowed.

CHAPTER 12

ONE THOUSAND COWS

"*...*Uh, uh...one thousand cows...one thousand cows...." Hervey mumbled.

He was just coming back to consciousness after having his second seizure in the emergency room. The head of the bed was up and the nurse was standing over him. She gave him something to stop any more seizures for now. She propped his head to prevent him from swallowing his tongue or choking on his own spit.

"What is he talking about? One thousand cows?" I asked.

"You mean like one thousand times. That is how many times I have seen him in the emergency room over the last two years. Sometimes he was here three or four times a day. It was always something. He would not take the prescription medications to control the seizures. Every time I checked the blood work the level for the medication was zero."

"Hervey, you are not taking the medication I gave you for seizures. What's the problem?"

I knew that he had a mental health problem but he just would not go to the psychiatrist where I had sent him. The last time he was here I begged the psychiatrist to give him another appointment. Now it made three times that he had not shown up for the visit. How many more times should you waste for him to take another person's appointment and don't show up? There were many other people needing to see her, so why should she bother with someone who was not ready or willing to be helped? Hervey also had a primary care doctor that he very well could have gone to for treatment.

Hey, Hervey. You might as well get a job in the emergency room, as you would have better work attendance than some of us. Every time I turned around he was here. It was like Pavlov's theory and the dog. The theory was that dogs repeat behavior because of how they are rewarded or punished. With Pavlov's experiment, he gave the dog a treat for good behavior and that reinforced it. After the dog behaved in a way that Pavlov did not want, the dog was punished. In time the dog knew what to expect and what to do. It was the same as with a child and a hot stove. You did it once and got burned. You did not go back to be burned over and over again, unless you could not learn. What was it about Hervey? Were we rewarding Hervey each time he came in the emergency room? Or was there some mental health problem that prevented him from connecting and remembering what happened before?

I was only the doctor in the emergency room, and not his family, but this was the last straw. I was feeling frustrated therefore I only imagined what his family felt.

"Hervey," I said. "You have a problem. Go to the psychiatrist. You either have depression, anxiety, another type of mental health problem, posttraumatic stress disorder, or a traumatic brain injury. But something is not right."

"I even gave you the peer support group number for you to call. They will help by talking to you when you don't feel well and feel like you need to come to the emergency room. They will help you to remember to take the seizure medications."

But, he didn't follow up with the peer support group. In fact, the last time when he called for help and said he was home, when they got there he was not.

"You also know that you have to stop drinking alcohol and smoking marijuana. It is like adding fuel to the fire. You will not get better this way."

addiction

I felt like his family and was wringing my own wrists in anguish. I wondered if he was doing this intentionally. He burned every bridge and the people who supported him. Whenever his name came up people would roll their eyes and get a glaze over their faces.

We needed to find a better way because I thought about the time and money spent over the last three years taking care of him. If he did not stick to a plan and find out what the underlying problem was, we could be doing this for many years. I had already admitted him too many times to count. The last time he was on a medical ward which was not a locked unit. He was admitted by his own free will, but when he felt better, in the midst of everything, he just got up and left against medical advice. I could not say that he was mentally incompetent to manage his affairs, at least not yet.

I remember when I was doing my psychiatry rotation in medical school. For six weeks I was on a locked psychiatric ward to learn the psychiatric diagnoses and the different kinds of persons living with mental illness. I walked up to the locked steel door with the squared pane of glass where you could see through to the other side. I rang the buzzer for the nurses to let me in, and no sooner had I entered than the door slammed shut.

 The first couple of days there I was nervous and overwhelmed by the number of men and women walking around. Not everyone was disheveled or having a conversation with themselves. Many of them were in different stages of recovery, were interacting appropriately with others, and ready to move on to the next phase of their lives and rejoin their community. One of the things that struck me was the need to be seen as a good person. Because, even the patients who were psychotic and thought they were someone else never said they were a person with a bad reputation. I met patients who said they were Jesus Christ, Joan of Arc, Martin Luther King or Gandhi. I even met Elvis, Bob Marley, and Einstein. None of these patients ever said they were any characters from history that had a bad reputation.

Therefore, from my perspective, I felt that even when they were living with mental illness, there was some intense need to be seen as a good person. And something was missing in the brain structure and chemicals that took them off course from being the kind of person they really wanted to be. When they did the "bad" things, when they were better, they did not remember any of the bad things that you told them they had done.

I wanted to believe that Hervey wanted to get better. I spoke to him sternly to stop drinking and stop using marijuana. None of that talking seemed to help. I met his elderly mother and I knew that she had her own health issues. After a while, I am sure she was simply exhausted. She could not keep up with the constant care that he needed. Where could she turn for help? There were family support groups in the city. But at the end of the day, she was it. In the midst of the multiple crises you get tired. I learned that you cannot do this alone, and it takes a team of people to deal with this lifelong problem.

I knew because I was living through that same pain at home but could not talk about it. Sam had been hospitalized for more than a year in the mental institution. I went often and my mother went practically every day. It was a good thing that Russell, Esther's brother, was able to drive her there. She was eternally grateful to him for doing that.

I was torn. I wanted to have a life. Esther wanted to have a life too. Was there a way for us to find balance?

Cabana Boy

Every now and then I had to remind myself that I had volunteered for this work. But there were times I felt like I was a cabana boy. I had to help Sam with all his daily activities. I had to help him in the shower, lay his clothes out, and clean up his room. I felt like I was on constant call. But, whenever I started to feel down about it, I looked at the good side. Sam was not homeless, out on the streets. His mental state was good. Sure, there were ups and downs and every now and then he had to be in the hospital. That was life. I had learned a lot about myself and I learned a lot about patience. I had signed up for this and no one had forced me to do it.

The trick though was to not be an enabler. I had to make Sam do the things that I knew he was able to do by himself, and not always depend on me to do everything.

That time when I cleaned out the room at the residential program where he was staying, some of the staff said I was an enabler. There was that fine line that you walked, but I did not make it a tightrope. If I worried about every opinion that someone had I would never be happy. I tried to make right choices. Some I got right, some I didn't. If my watch fell into the sea while swimming, so be it. I left it there. Time did not wait for anyone and I did not feel like wasting time worrying about a mistake I had made. I learned from the mistake and moved on.

I didn't want to wallow in self-pity, and Esther never liked a sob story. But neither of us could sleep well at night knowing that Sam was living on the streets. If it required a little bit of sacrifice, then so be it. But, I would be lying if I told you that at times that I did not feel resentful. But, I found a way to enjoy each day and to be hopeful. It was not always, up, up, up…but I laughed a lot and cried a lot and allowed myself just to be me.

TIP BOX 3

1. Don't be voiceless: Speak up for what you believe is right. There are family advocates and peer support groups who can help you do this if you are not able to do this on your own

2. Ask for the right help: Use a team that includes health professionals, community resources, family, and good friends

3. Volunteer in your community: Help someone else along the way. You will find that it helps to give your own life meaning

PART IV

EYE OF THE STORM

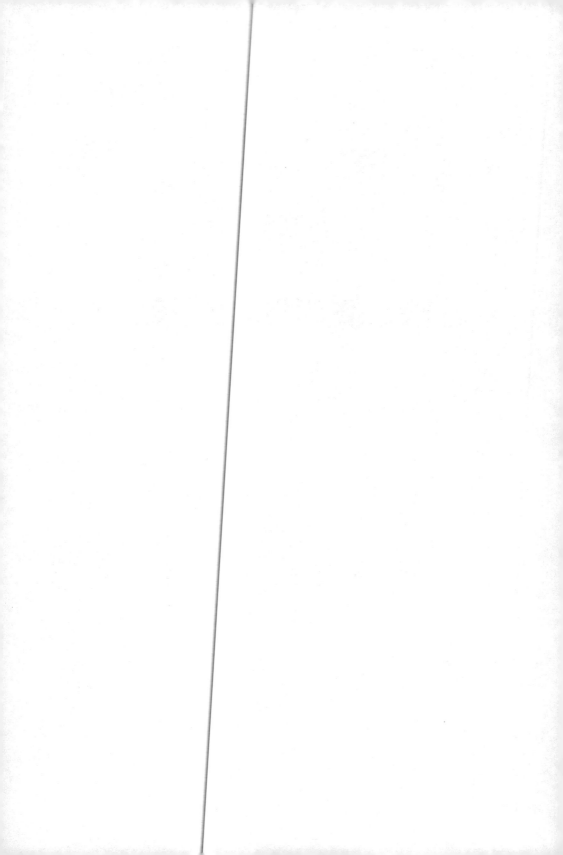

Different, by Donna Wilkinson Maxwell

For as long as I can remember
I knew you were different,
As children growing up
You were just so distant.
There was a problem we could not understand
But it seemed much greater
Certainly not what we had planned
But there was no other, my blood... my brother.
Then different became belligerent
We did not know what to do
It must be a discipline problem,
That's what they said to us at school.
This was more than we could manage
We had no idea how to build that bridge and stop all the damage
But still there was no other, my blood…my brother.
You grew up and left home
You took to the streets and there you roamed.
We could not help you, we only faced defeat
So we left you to walk the beat.
Your actions were not intentional,
You just needed some help
You were actually institutional
We didn't know it then.
You couldn't do it by yourself
Still yet there was no other, my blood…my brother.

Although it is difficult and certainly not grand,
I've taken you under my roof
To lend a helping hand
You can take comfort that I'll do my best
So you can have shelter, peace and rest.
At times I'll need to rejuvenate
Regain my strength so I can relate
Have a clear mind to handle this task
Which I do freely, you don't have to ask.
With confidence I can say,
There is no other, my blood…my brother.

CHAPTER 13

MISSION IMPOSSIBLE

we want freedom

I only wanted to be free.

Sam wanted to be free too to have hope for a brighter day and not to be in the eye of the storm with mental illness.

I had watched Tom Cruise scale the Burj Khalifa in the movie, *Mission: Impossible - Ghost Protocol,* and envisioned the day when Sam would have his mind back for a long time. I longed for the day when he would be free from the burden of feeling helpless and hopeless. The Khalifa was in Dubai and was now the tallest building and the tallest free-standing structure in the world. Dubai was now a thriving city in the middle of a desert where the people found a fertile spot and built a life there. They created canals bringing in more water to help tame a parched land.

I looked at the skyline of Dubai filled with skyscrapers gently touching eternity. In only a few decades Dubai had transformed itself from a tiny fishing village on the Dubai Creek to a world class city with state-of-the-art amenities and was a popular tourist destination. For me, it was like living and breathing in my lifetime a transformation that all great cities go through, as New York; Washington, D.C.; Beijing; London; Nairobi; and Tokyo had.

mind is not free when caregiving

How does one even imagine the possibility of such greatness when all you see around you is desert sand and no water? How do you quench your thirst for sanity and a mind that is free to enjoy your life? How do you do it? How did Dubai do it?

Somewhere along the line I had become complacent. I gave Sam his medications every morning and every evening so I was convinced that he was taking them. Over a week or two I had not noticed the subtle changes where he was talking less and seemed withdrawn. He was like a robot. As soon as it came to five o'clock in the evening he wanted to go to his bedroom. He had me pull all the shades down in his room and that blocked out all the sunlight. Yikes, it was still sunny even up to 7 p.m., so why lay there in the darkness?

At one o'clock in the morning I had to go to his room to turn the television off as it was blasting all day. He was lying there in bed and I assumed he was sleeping but he wasn't. After one more day of him being withdrawn, he became more irritable and demanding. Everything had to be done now, STAT. If I was in the middle of getting myself a cup of coffee or reading the newspaper he would come up to me to ask for something that was not even needed.

"Hey, can it wait until I am done?" I asked

"No. I need that now," he said.

"OK, wait until when I shave you," I said.

"No, I don't want a shave or a haircut," he said.

"Did you shower today, or yesterday for that matter?"

"Yes, I showered this morning," he mumbled.

Well, I knew that was a big lie. I had cleaned the bath tub this morning and it might have well been a desert. There was not an ounce of water anywhere. I sniffed the early sweet apple rot of two days body odor. I tried to ignore him and avoided the signs. Intuition means to be taught from within, information that you have inside you but sometimes choose to ignore for whatever reason. But, I wanted to be free and my mind was not free.

The next morning I came down stairs to the kitchen very early and I heard a rustling that should not have been there. Esther was not up and I had not left any machines on there. I had slept like a log from the exhaustion from running around in the emergency room.

Sam had a knife in his hand.

"I want to kill myself," he said.

What the hell? Who left that knife there? I always scanned the kitchen before going to bed and hid any sharp knives.

"I want to end it now! I am going to die this year and it is time!"

"Put the knife down, Sam."

"Give me the knife, Sam."

"No, I want to die. I can't live this way."

"I can't live anymore!"

He held the knife up and made as if to slash his left wrist. Was it only a gesture, a cry for help? Would I get a warning sign when he really meant it? Should I not have seen this day coming? How did I miss the signs?

"Put the knife down, Sam. Put the knife down."

"Sam, put the knife down now, now, put the knife down."

I had missed the signs and was distracted by wanting to have my own life. I had volunteered for this work so what was I complaining about? When Sam was younger, Esther had grabbed the scissors out of his hand when he chopped off all of his hair in the bathroom. I wasn't naïve. Many family members get injured trying to take a weapon away from a family member trying to kill themselves. I also worked in the emergency room and knew to remove all contraband from patients who are suicidal, homicidal or just in a bad place mentally. I had to let him put the knife down so that I could grab it and call the ambulance. I had learned to de-escalate crisis situations, speak in a calm voice but not to put myself in harm's way.

"Sam, I am here with you. Put the knife down and let's talk about it. You are not alone. We can make it if we do this together."

"Put the knife down."

Sam placed the knife on the counter and I quickly snatched it up. I stepped forward and pulled the portable phone off its base and called 911. There were no other sharp objects around and I told Sam to stand there for a minute and I jogged to the front door to open it wide. That way when the police came with the ambulance I could call them in and not go back to the door. They had been here before, so maybe it was someone who knew the house and had some idea of the situation. The police arrived before the ambulance, but it too arrived within minutes.

"Sam, you have to go to the hospital."

"I am right there with you. Go with them in the ambulance and I will drive behind them."

The presence of other people, the police and the ambulance crew, was helpful as now I was not alone. I really needed a team just to have a physical presence even if they just stood there quietly. It had a calming effect on me and on Sam as well. The ambulance took Sam out and drove him to the emergency room. That was the beginning of another long hospitalization for Sam to control his schizophrenia and bipolar depression.

I had only wanted to be free, and in that need lost focus on why I was here, and on what I was doing. When you are flying in an airplane the flight attendants also tell you that in an emergency if the plane loses cabin pressure, you need to put your oxygen mask on first before you can help others around. If you can't breathe you can't help others. No one wants to come onto a sinking ship either. I volunteered. I had to make sure that my ship was not sinking and if it started to take on water, I needed to be alert enough to dump it out, and toss all the burdens and unnecessary items that made me sink. Sam needed a stable ship. If I were to help, I had to be anchored myself; otherwise, we would both go down to the bottomless pit.

Dubai created the Burj Khalifa in the middle of a desert, and it was designed to withstand the worse storms and horrific wind forces. Cruise scaled it in an impossible mission. I dreamed of walking into that building one day to go to the tippy top and look out and look forward. If we can create that in the middle of a desert, what is there in life that cannot be overcome? To dream the impossible dream, to plan for it and actually live it out in real life. I vowed to get Sam out of the eye of the storm and create a day when we could enjoy sunny skies. To get there though, there would be days of rain and calm after the storm.

Parasites Roosting

When Sam was floridly psychotic, he would have periods when he would tell you some bizarre things. The thought problems associated with schizophrenia are known as psychosis. Sometimes, Sam's thinking was completely out of touch with reality. What he was telling you certainly could not be real. Sam would insist that there were bugs, spiders, or tarantulas crawling in his skin.

In order not to rock the boat and simply say outright that these things are all in your mind, and not real, I would unwillingly oblige him and take a look at his skin. I looked at his arms and back and trunk and thighs. I almost knew for certain each time that I looked that I would find nothing, but I looked anyway. With a smile to reassure him, I triumphantly said, "look, Sam, there are no bugs on your skin." However, this rarely reassured him.

"See there is one now," he responded. I would look to where he was pointing and I saw nothing. As time went on I began to doubt myself. Maybe there were insects on his skin and body that I could not see. Maybe it was time for me to get my eyes checked. I turned him around, lifted his shirt. Nothing. Well, if bugs were there, I should be able to see a tarantula with my bare eyes. I adjusted my glasses. I still did not see anything. No bug or insect was there and I knew it. Of course, I knew no bug or insect was there. I don't even think those insects lived in this part of the world.

"There is nothing on your skin, or coming out of your skin," I said.

"Yes, there is," Sam said.

"Look again, you'll see," he insisted.

So, I was glad to be startled when my cell phone rang. This time it was Elizabeth with the same complaint. I thought, please no, here we go again.

"I feel like there are bugs crawling in me," she said.

"I am coming out of my skin!" Elizabeth exclaimed.

I liked the blue bird song quality of her voice. She was prone to hyperbole and melodrama, so I kept calm and thought, okay. Now, she too has bugs coming out of her skin too? Was it in the air or in the water? She had said "skin" with a higher squeaky tone and with so much emphasis that I could sense the feeling of whatever she thought was coming out or crawling on her skin. I squirmed and twisted to get the bugs out of me as well. Reflexively, I started to scratch at my own skin. There were no bugs or insects on me or in me. But, I kept on scratching my own skin in the hopes of creating an exit for the bugs to come out. I was experiencing what she was describing except that I did not understand what she meant.

"What do you mean?" I asked.

"I feel like I am coming out of my skin. I can't really explain it."

"Well, do you see a bug?"

"No. But I feel them."

"Do you have a rash? Do you see any tracks of anything that might have crawled on you? Well, is it that your skin is just itchy? Maybe, you are having some kind of skin irritation, like an allergic reaction? You can get an allergic reaction from contact with something new, something that you may not have been exposed to before. Did you start using a new product? Are you using any new medications?" I insisted.

I doubt there were bugs crawling on her body and skin. Elizabeth was a neat freak. She was always nicely dressed and she wore the latest styles and everything was well coordinated. I doubt that she had traveled anywhere recently. And knowing her she probably would have rented a bedbug sniffing dog to sniff out the beds and chairs before she would sit or sleep in the bed. She would boast that the first thing she did when she went into a hotel room was to remove all the spreads and covers. At times, before she would even sit on the bed she would insist that housekeeping bring her up new sheets and pillow cases. If they would not and time allowed, she would to go a department store and buy new sheets and pillows. More often than not, she had already brought a set of sheets and pillowcases with her from home anyway. She would simply change the linens before she laid her head and body on any of it.

I had resigned myself to live without fear of bugs or insects. In fact, I trained myself to not have much fear of anything. That was especially true if I could not see or touch it. If the source of the potential fear was not tangible then I would not become as fastidious as to become paranoid about something that I could not see or touch. Some supreme power had given humankind the knowledge for us to make Kwell and Rid and insect sprays. In fact, the power had given us the knowledge so that we could prevent sickness and death from many microbes.

I wanted to say, "Elizabeth, get Kwell and forget-about-it!" But of course, I could not say that as she was in distress.

"Okay, any new soaps, powders, cosmetics, sheets? A new cat, dog or pet? Anything new, any new exposures?" I asked.

"No."

"Well, did you travel?"

She said that she had not left the city or state and that there were no new changes that she could immediately think of.

"You don't see the bug, insect or parasite?" I asked.

"No. None. I don't see it. But, I know it's there."

Well, I thought, don't go down that line of reasoning with her. You are not there. You cannot observe to see if there is a bug on her skin or not.

"So," I said instead, "well, it could be a problem with your kidney or liver."

"Have you gone to your doctor for an exam and advice?"

"Maybe, what you are describing has something to do with something else. You should make an appointment to see your doctor and have your doctor check," I said again.

"Well, I went to the doctor before and she did not find anything wrong with my blood work."

"Really? But you may still want to go this time since this is a new episode and something has changed," I said.

Yes, that sounds like what Sam would say—that he went to the doctors, they checked everything and found nothing. Sometimes, he said the bug or insect or parasite or foreign object was coming out of his entire body. Is that what Elizabeth was saying?

"I feel parasites roosting," Sam proclaimed. "Parasites are coming out of me. Somebody is coming out of me. Parasites roosting," he said.

"Let me see," I said again.

I would look carefully again over his body. I did not see a rash. I did not see any irritations. There was nothing on his body that looked like a parasite was roosting. There was nothing that looked like scabies. It was highly unlikely that he had picked up a bed bug. Just like Elizabeth, he hardly traveled. He had not been sleeping in any usual places, at least not lately. He had not been homeless and living on the streets for a while now.

"I don't see anything," I declared to him.

"Well, I feel 'icky,'" he said.

"Huh," I said and made a mental note to continue to observe his behaviors and call Dr. Bernard to discuss what I was observing and hearing. But, was Elizabeth saying that? Was that the same thing? Was she saying that non-existent parasites were coming out of her body? I did not know her to have a mental illness with any delusional qualities. Then I thought how would you really know? I had known Elizabeth for thirty years. Last week

I heard her sing in a beautiful soprano at a church service. She had sung "The Lighthouse." I was blown away by her beautiful rendition and sat there thinking —"You must be kidding me. I have known you all these years and have never heard you sing."

"Wow, amazing," I said to myself. I never heard her singing, and if I had, I certainly had not heard her sing like that. In fact, if anyone asked me if Elizabeth could sing, I would say, "Of course not, in fact, I think she is tone deaf, she cannot even carry a tune." Yet, last week when she sang I was stunned into silence.

"I feel like I am coming out of my skin," she repeated.

She was not known to be psychotic or delusional. I had not known her to be hospitalized for any mental illness or behavioral health problem. What exactly was she describing? My mind raced trying to listen, to observe, and to narrow down the possibilities of what was the problem from what Elizabeth was describing. What exactly was the problem here?

Symptoms — how do we decide if they are mental illness?

CHAPTER 14

TELL BRET

I reached into my left lab-coat pocket and pulled out my personal cell phone. I wanted to use my own phone to make this call. I had the hospital's mobile phone in my right pocket. I balanced the phones with the pens and papers in the pockets to prevent the coat from loping to one side. I speed dialed Bret's number and he picked up on the second ring.

"Bret, can you help us?" I asked.

"What?" Bret asked.

"Can you help us?" I repeated. Had Bret lost his hearing?

"You know everybody and I am sure you can help. Bret, you know everybody. Call someone who can help us. Tell them we need to talk to them," I said.

Bret said nothing.

"Bret, are you listening? Did you hear anything of what I just said?" I asked. "Call someone, Bret, we need help."

"What's going on?" Bret asked.

"Seven people shot," I said. "Seven."

"When did that happen?" Bret asked.

"They are out there shooting up people. Just shooting randomly into a crowd of people. There was a shooting at the celebration parade. Shooting into a crowd at a parade. Who does that? Are we at war? Is this a war zone, Bret?" I asked.

"What?" Bret asked again. He apparently had not heard me. Was he even listening to anything that I had just said?

"Did you not hear what I just said?" I asked. "Seven people shot. I just had to intubate a seven year old boy as he was shot in the head. This is terrible," I said. "We don't have the time for this."

"Now the hospital is in lock down. Nobody can come in and nobody can go out. The police are all over the place. All the city police are here and I am sure there is not one police left on the streets."

"Is this what we have come to? Are we living in a war zone right smack in the middle of the city?" I asked.

Only minutes before the red emergency phone had gone off. The paramedics had called and said that there was a shooting at the annual parade. They were bringing in the victim, or victims.

"Oh, we will give you the report and update when we come in," they said.

"Could you tell us anything else, anything more?" One of the nurses had asked them.

"Nope. We do not have any more information at this point," was the response.

"Should it be a Full Trauma or a Core Trauma?" I asked when the nurse came to tell me.

"What are we expecting?" I asked.

"Dr. Gary, look, I have no idea. Not a clue. I don't know," she shrugged and said.

"Well, call a Full Trauma," I said. "That way we are fully prepared. We can always downgrade the trauma call if we do not need a full court press."

The nurse had called the hospital operator to tell her to call a Full Trauma Code. Immediately, the page went over head to call the code. Good. That way the on-call trauma team will come running to the trauma room. I ran to the blue bin outside the trauma room and grabbed a paper gown out and let the others fall back in. It was one size fits-all. I put latex gloves on and went into the trauma room. What was going on? Now there is a shooting at the parade right smack in broad daylight?

It seemed like it took an eternity for the paramedics to arrive but in reality hardly five minutes had gone by. The ambulance arrived at the loading area and I waited in the trauma room. Had they call back to give us an update? If they had I had not heard it. What was coming in? What were we to expect? Was it one victim or more than one? Would we be ready?

You have to be ready in the emergency room and I was ready for anything. But, curiosity was getting the best of me, therefore, as I had the gown and gloves on, I popped out of the room and jogged the short distance to the ambulance bay. I wanted to meet the stretcher. What was it that they were going to serve up now?

Out of habit I would have waited by the door to the trauma room. I would place myself at the head of the stretcher as I was in charge of the airway and this was the best position to wait in. Know your ABCs. I had to get the A correct otherwise there would be no B or C. The A was to manage the airway. If needed, I would have to intubate the patient if there were any problems with breathing. All the airway supplies were at the top end of the room. The trauma room was organized in this way so that all the supplies and equipment needed for the top half of the body was here. All the other equipment needed to treat the lower half of the body was at the opposite end of the room. There had to be order among the chaos.

The paramedics were hurriedly trying to get the stretcher off the ambulance. I was next to them in a flash.

"Huh?" I muttered.

There was a small clump of sheets on the stretcher, but otherwise it looked empty. Is this it? What was going on? Is this it?

"Where is the patient? Why are you rushing? Where is the patient?" I asked. "Where is the patient?"

"Dr. Gary," the paramedic said.

"Doc. Doc. It's a kid. It's a kid. He has been shot in the head. It's a kid, it's a kid."

"Tray," I shouted back to anyone listening in the trauma room.

"Get the Pedi tray. Get the pediatric tray, now. " I yelled back to the trauma room. I flung myself around and ran back with the crew to the trauma room.

Purity, the nurse assigned to the trauma room for this shift, came running with the pediatric intubation tray. She stopped at my side and quickly ripped away the sterile covering from the tray. Purity was from Ethiopia but she had been living in the United States for over five years. Purity. I always thought that was an odd name. Purity. Well, I guess it is better than being named "Internet." What would be the meaning behind naming your child that?

"Did you get an IV? Did you get an intravenous line in?" I asked the paramedic.

"Yes, at least we got that in. Yes. I got one in his right arm," he sputtered.

"We did not have time to "tube" him. There was no time to intubate him," he apologized. He was breathing heavily and kept on saying "we did not have time to tube him, there was no time, doc."

"Everything happened so fast. We just grabbed him and ran," he said.

"Excellent," I said. "Excellent, you got an IV in. No problem. We will take care of it."

"Purity, prepare the meds," I said. "Have the atropine on standby just in case his pulse goes too low" I added, and Purity nodded.

"Purity? Also grab the calibrated pediatric tape and place it on the bed by the boy's head so that way we can estimate his height and weight. That will help us dose the medications correctly," I added. Purity was ahead as she had already placed the board on the stretcher by the boy. I gave the medication orders to Purity. Ryan and Hope were busy taking down notes and documenting all that was happening in the room. The paramedics continued talking to give their report and I listened and worked at the same time. The boy was shot while standing with his father at the parade. The shooting appeared to be random into the crowd. Rigoberto, a paramedic, said no, it was not random.

"It was meant for a specific target," Rigoberto said. "Of course, this child and six others just happened to be in the shooter's way," he said.

"There are six more persons shot?" I asked Rigoberto. I was still looking into the boy's mouth and airway.

"Did they call those reports of other persons coming in?" I asked.

"What? Are you kidding?" I asked, now wondering if sufficient staff was readily available.

"We did not get a report that this was a pediatric trauma with a gunshot wound. No one said that this was a gunshot wound to the head," I said in disbelief. "Now you are saying there are more victims?" I asked.

"We needed to know that information so that we are prepared," I said.

"More victims? Are they all coming here?" I asked.

"Ryan. Call the charge nurse now. Let the other doctors in the emergency room and the surgeons know what's going on. We need all hands on deck. They all need to come to help. Tell them to stop seeing other patients. We need their help."

"Call emergency medical services and ask what else is coming in. We need to know so that we can get ready," I said. We were not in a war zone. Or were we? Everything else had to be on stand-by. "Let the charge nurse and doctors know," I said again.

The nurses placed the boy on the monitor to track the blood pressure and his heart rate. A pulse oximeter monitored the level of oxygen in the blood. I stood over the head of the bed directly above the young boy's head. God, he was young. He appeared to be only about six or seven years old. I watched the rising and falling of his chest. He was breathing. Good, at least he is breathing. Standing at the head of the bed I could see that his mouth was free of blood. There were no injuries to the mouth, face or throat but the boy was not talking and he had his eyes closed.

"Open your eyes," I said. "Open your eyes."

I did not want to pry the boy's eyes open to look at them. Was he even awake? Would he follow my voice? Were his eyes closed because he was in pain? Or was there a severe head injury that caused him to be unconscious? He did not respond to my voice but, he was breathing.

"Bring the light to check his pupils," I said to one of the surgical residents.

"We need to intubate him," I said.

"With this gunshot head injury, we need to "tube" him," I said. "That bullet could be anywhere in his head and we need to get him into the CAT scan like super STAT," I said.

I uncovered the bandage that the crew had placed over the right side of the boy's head. Once the bandage was removed I was looking into a hole in the skull where the blood was coming from and trickling through the gauze. The blood stained his head, the sheets and the stretcher. The jagged entrance wound of the bullet was near the side of his temple and was about two inches immediately upwards from his right ear. I did not see where the bullet came out on the other side. The paramedics had fixed the boy's neck with a small plastic cervical collar. Since there was no exit the bullet was lodged somewhere in his head. I put an oxygen mask closer to the boy's face.

"Purity, give the medicines now," I said.

In less than a minute, the boy stopped breathing, and I slid the curved blade into the middle of his mouth. I avoided hitting his teeth, and I slid the blade quickly to the back of his tongue. I lifted the soft palate so that I could see the epiglottis that covered the path to his airway. I advanced the blade into the groove behind the epiglottis to expose the vocal cords which did not move. The medication had also stopped the vocal cords from moving. Simultaneously, as I was advancing the blade, I had been sliding the tube forward. I had held it in my left hand, and moved the tube along the left side of his mouth. Once I saw the epiglottis and lifted it, I made the last movement to put the tube into the upper trachea. I held onto the tube, and moved the upper tip over to the side of his mouth. I attached the Ambu bag to it to give him oxygen. I squeezed the Ambu bag twice to get the oxygen into the boy's lungs, and I looked to see the rise and fall of his chest. I bent slightly forward, and placed my stethoscope into my ear. I had to slightly contort myself as I was holding the tube with my left hand. I placed the right ear-piece of the stethoscope in my right ear with my right hand. The stethoscope's upper metal bar twisted on my face as the left handle caught on my left cheek. Remina, the respiratory tech beside me, tried to help to put the left ear-piece in my left ear but, it was too much out of her way. She would have to bend past the ventilator, as it stood in the way immediately to my right at the bedside. I changed hands, and held the tube with my right hand, and then placed the left ear-piece into my left ear. That was much better as my ears would have been torn apart if I had kept the left handle of the stethoscope on my left cheek any longer. The right ear-piece was already in my right ear. If I had not moved quickly, I would have been strangled by the plastic portion of the stethoscope.

Now that the tube was in its correct position, I listened over the boy's chest. The breath sounds were equal over both lungs. I listened over his stomach as well. I did not hear any muffled sounds of air there when I squeezed the bag. That was good. I had not placed the tube into his esophagus, and passing the oxygen into his stomach which was not where it needed to be. I was confident that the tube was already in its rightful place. However, I had to confirm the tube's correct placement by going through the necessary steps. Remina placed the carbon dioxide monitor between the tube and the Ambu bag, and she pumped the Ambu bag once to make his lungs expand. The carbon dioxide monitor changed color verifying that the tube was correctly placed in the airway. The oxygen saturation monitor showed a normal reading.

"Good," I said. We had done all the steps to document the correct placement of the tube into the airway.

"Dr. Gary, I will take over now. Let me secure the tube with tape and put him on the vent. You can go do something else," Remina said.

"Great," I said. I moved from around the ventilator and ducked to prevent hitting my head on the large overhead monitor. Remina could secure the tube and put the boy on the vent.

"What vent settings do you want?" Remina asked.

"The usual," I said. "After he is stable Luke and his team can get blood work and then you can change the settings as needed," I said. Ryan was the recording nurse so he put all of that information on the trauma flow sheet.

"Okay, Luke," I said.

"He is all yours. Work your magic. He is all set to go to the CAT scan suite."

"We need to know where that bullet in his head lodged," I said. "Oh, take sedatives and muscle relaxants with you when you go to CAT scan as those medicines will wear off soon. You don't want him to wake up and feel that tube in his mouth."

Hope walked quickly back into the trauma room and she had a worried look on her face.

"Yes. Six more were shot. Three more are coming here," Hope said.

"The other hospital will take the other three."

"Huh," I said. I was speechless and no more words could come out after I had heard what she had just said.

"One is critical and shot in the chest," Hope said.

"The paramedics have "tubed" him in the field and they should be here any minute now. We will see what else we have when they get here," she said.

"We can put him in the next room. Once they take the boy to CAT scan, you can take that new one. We will get the other doctors to run the other two traumas," Hope said.

"Good, that will work," I said.

Dr. Luke Jones and his team had done their exam, the boy was stable, and they could take him to CAT scan. Hopefully, he would remain stable and the get entire scan done. The respiratory tech and Dr. Jones were just about to leave the trauma room when the next victim came in.

"Dr. Gary, I will take this one for you. I see that you already have your hands full," Dr. Lipson said as he came into the trauma room.

"Great, do that, he's all yours," I said. Between the two patients, I had no time to pull off my gown or gloves from working with the boy. So I welcomed Dr. Lipson's help. I would have had to rip off one gown and gloves, wash my hands, and then gown and glove back up. I had no time to do any of that.

"Yes, please take this one. Besides, there is a call I must make," I said. I stepped out of the trauma room, and I pulled off the gown and gloves. When I reached the nearest sink I washed my hands, and dried them with paper towels. That was the point at which I had reached into the left lab-coat pocket to speed-dial Bret.

"Bret? Are you listening? Call somebody. Anybody," I said.

"The hospital is in lock down," I said.

"Are you hearing me? Are you hearing me, Bret?" I asked again.

Bret was in his own world. Earlier in morning he had called to ask my opinion about what to do about a situation. He said that he had been asleep early Friday morning when at one o'clock in the morning his cell phone rang. He awoke, dazed at first. He was confused as he was awakening from a very deep sleep. It was Agnes, his assistant, who was on his cell phone at that time of the morning.

"Bret," she said, "I won't be at work in the morning."

"Why, Agnes?" Bret asked.

"Phillip, you know, my son, has gotten into the medicine cabinet, you know," Agnes said.

"Uh, uh," Bret said.

"Well, he got into the laxatives," Agnes said.

"Okay?" Bret said.

"Yeah, he got into the laxatives. You know how boys are. He took more than a handful of them, and now he's having diarrhea," Agnes said.

"So, I won't be at work in the morning," Agnes repeated.

"Okay?" Bret asked again. What was he to do? What was he to say, or what was he to ask?

"Maybe you should take him to the hospital to make sure he is okay?" Bret asked.

"No," Agnes said. "He is not vomiting."

"He is only having diarrhea. You know, I can't take him to the babysitter today like this. So, I have to stay home with him. I have to make sure he is okay," Agnes said.

"It's Friday. It's the weekend. Tomorrow is Saturday. I think he will be okay. I will watch him and see how he does. If he gets worse I will take him to the emergency room. He is not vomiting, so I think he will be okay. See you on Monday, Bret. I will not be at work today."

"Uh, sure. Okay then," Bret said. The call ended and he fell back to sleep. He called me when he woke up later in the day on Friday morning.

"What should I do? Should I report her to DCF?"

"Whoa. Where did that come from? What makes you think you need to make a report to the Department of Children and Families? Do you think that Agnes is abusing her child?"

"Did she give her son the laxatives on purpose?"

"Do you think she gave Phillip the laxatives intentionally to make him have diarrhea? Do you think that she would do that so she can call you at one in the morning? Just to say she can't come to work? Would she really do that?" I pressed him some more.

"I mean, she wouldn't have to give Phillip the laxative and then call you as a work excuse, right? Anyway, she could be lying. You wouldn't even know if Phillip took any laxative and was having diarrhea or not. So she could call you and tell you anything and you would not know the difference. I don't think that is the problem. Do you suspect that she is abusing her son at all? I mean, child abuse could be physical, emotional or sexual. It could even be by withholding food and meals. Was she starving her child? Have you ever even seen him?" I asked Bret.

"Have you ever seen him with bruises or cuts or injuries? Did you ever see Phillip with anything that looked unusual or an explanation of an injury that did not make sense? Was the explanation inconsistent and did not make sense for the age of the child and his motor development?"

"Does it seem as if Agnes is not taking care of her son?" I pushed Bret to explain.

"Is Phillip not properly clothed? Does he look dirty, hungry or poorly fed? You have seen him before, right?" I asked Bret. I was trying to figure out where he was coming from.

"You don't think this is an intentional ingestion, do you? I mean, hey. Maybe she won't win the parent of the year award. Maybe she could use some parenting classes. We probably all could use them. Hey, she should not have laxatives in a medicine cabinet where her son can reach them. Besides, isn't Phillip only like, three years old, if that?"

"Can he even walk?" I asked laughing. Bret was ridiculous to even think about Agnes' tale. Did she really tell him that or was he so asleep he had forgotten what she had told him. He had been half asleep. Does he even really remember the details of the conversation that he had with Agnes? Really, if she did not want to come to work why not just call in and say that she can't come to work? Why make up such a story? Why would she have to fabricate such a thing? Then again if it were true, why was it Bret's problem? I asked myself.

"How could her son reach the medicine cabinet to get into laxatives anyway?" I asked Bret.

"I mean is the child superman? Did he fly up to reach the medicine cabinet?" I asked Bret laughing much too loudly now. If the patients and my colleagues in the emergency room were hearing my side of the conversation, and heard me laughing so loudly they would have thought that I had lost a screw. Maybe the elevator was not going all the way to the top. I am sure they were thinking, "Doc must have lost it."

"No. I did not ask her all of that," Bret said.

"I hate talking to you," Bret said in exasperation.

"Why's that?" I asked still laughing.

"Because, you always ask too many questions," Bret said. "It's like the third degree. It's like you're *Perry Mason* or somebody."

"*Perry Mason*?" I asked. "He is well before my time. Was I even born then? *Perry Mason,* for crying out loud. Who in creation would know him? Bret, you are so 'old-school.'"

"Anyway, Bret, *Perry Mason*? Wrong profession, wrong era. Wasn't *Perry Mason* a lawyer, an attorney? Maybe, you mean, like *Marcus Welby, MD*? Stick to the present Bret. Are you having memory loss? Are you having a break with reality? Do you mean inquisitive and curious like *House*? Do you mean like *Doctor House*?" I asked.

"I mean, wake up, Bret, are you still sleeping? Are you forgetting things? This is new-school now, buddy. The modern era. Wake up and smell the coffee. Or better yet, drink some, because you were obviously still asleep, Bret," I said. I laughed out again. Bret started to laugh too as he knew he had to get with the program.

"Bret," I said, "I am only asking because Agnes' story sounds just too unbelievable."

"She probably just did not want to go to work today," I said.

"I mean, who calls their boss at one o'clock in the morning to say their child got into some laxatives, has diarrhea, and that she can't come to work?" I asked. "Do you think she has Munchausen syndrome by proxy? Is she trying to get her child deliberately sick so that she can take him to the doctors? I mean, is she trying to fake a medical illness for her child? If you think that, Agnes probably would have a mental illness, right?" I asked.

"Well, you know, I was so asleep when she called and I don't even know if I got the story right. I was so asleep and confused that I could not think straight and ask any questions," Bret said.

"Well, don't get me wrong," I said. "She would not be the first parent with a mental illness raising a child. And that does not mean that even if she had a mental health problem that she will be a bad parent," I added. "Maybe something else is going on and the explanation is completely reasonable."

"Yeah, I know that. But, I thought that the situation was not right, and maybe I should report it to somebody," Bret said.

"It is probably something else. Such as, did you have some big project or work that you gave her to do? Maybe that alone will make her not want to come to work?" I asked.

"No, I did not give her anything like that," Bret answered.

"But she just finalized her divorce. I think she is going through a tough time," Bret added.

"Like, yeah!" I said. "It does sound like she has a lot going on and is just stressed out."

I remember when I had to ask Dr. Maurice, my supervisor and the director of the emergency room, if I could change my schedule to work only the weekend twelve-hour shifts and not work during the week. I was so stressed out from having Sam at home and working full-time hours at the same time. There are very few adult sitters around that will come into your house when you need them. Unless it is family you don't really get a break to simply run to the store or even to a movie. For the most part other family members are living their own lives working and taking care of their own problems. Even when there was an adult sitter most of the time they were not comfortable working with someone with a history of mental illness, even when that person was stable on their medications. They were fearful of them and they did not want to come back twice.

Occasionally, I used the adult daycare option, but if Sam did not want to go out that day then all my plans would need to be put on hold. I changed my schedule to be home during the week and worked on the weekends. It got to the point where I worked all weekends for three years and missed all the sports, concerts and other things that my friends were doing. When I had to ask for the schedule change I had to tell Maurice about my life, something that really wasn't his business. Why should he even care? But, no one liked working the weekends anyway, so the other doctors must have been glad to hear of it. In any case, I don't think I thought of calling Maurice in the morning to make up an excuse why I could not come to work.

"She probably just has a lot going on, and can't really tell you what it is. I bet she has some other problem," I said.

"Among them is calling you at one in the morning. She could just as well have called at eight in the morning. But that just sounds like an attendance and work related problem. You can figure that one out easily and deal with it," I said.

"But as for DCF, there is nothing that you have told me to make me think that getting into the laxatives was something that was done on purpose," I said.

"You don't have enough information to even suspect child abuse. So unless you are willing to dig some more and get more information from Agnes, it does not sound like a good idea to call anyone. And Bret, anyway you are not a mandated reporter, meaning you are not a health care provider, or school, or social worker, or law enforcement worker, that says you have to report suspected child abuse and have it investigated by DCF."

"Unless I am completely off base, I don't think you have enough information to even suspect it," I added.

"You may have someone who I question their judgment on many levels. But, I am not so sure that you have enough information to suspect child abuse," I said.

"Okay, okay, I will ask Agnes some more questions and then we can talk more."

So, when Bret saw that I was now calling again on Saturday, he was probably thinking that I was calling to follow up on the conversation from yesterday. I don't think he was ready for anyone screaming into his cell phone, and unfortunately, it was me on the call.

"I just had to intubate a six year old child that was shot in the head" I said. My voice was twisted and rising in pain as I imagined what the pain would be like from being shot. But this was not a time to become overly emotional. I had to think through this calmly and logically. I needed Bret to act and act fast. I needed him to get me someone's telephone number. They needed to know the urgency of the situation. The community could not wait another day for talks and discussions and no progress. We needed to act and to act fast.

Just then Dr. Lipson stormed out of the trauma room. He ripped off the blue sterile paper gown and tossed his gloves into the nearest garbage can that he saw. He stomped off in the direction of the other rooms to pick up the work with his other patients. He had not been in the trauma bay for more than five minutes. He glared in my direction and made a horizontal hang man noose sign across his neck. He was showing me that the patient with the gunshot wound to the chest did not make it and had died.

Lipson walked over to tell me what the scene was like in the trauma room. Lipson was hardly five feet two inches tall but he was strapping and solidly built. He was a scholar-athlete. Not much of anything fazed him. He started his surgical training to be a heart surgeon, and did that training for two to three years. But, in middle of that training, he changed course and became an emergency room doctor instead. He had been working in the emergency room for more than twenty years. Like most of us who worked here, he was used to stress, uncertainty, and working with multiple traumas. He had seen his share of bodily injuries, mutilations, death, and disasters in general.

"Seven people shot," Lipson said in disgust. I nodded in agreement without saying anything.

"That young man died. He barely looked like twenty years old," Lipson said.

"Wow," I said to Lipson. "Unbelievable!"

"Yes. DOA. Dead on Arrival. The man had been shot in the chest. The paramedics intubated him at the scene, but, he had no blood pressure and no pulse while there. The crew tried to resuscitate him in the ambulance and gave him all the medications that they could before they got here. I was just calling for uncrossed blood but, it was no use. Dead on Arrival. Now, I have to go tell his family," Lipson said.

There were to be no heroics today. When the patient has a very slim chance of survival you still do all that you can to give them a fighting chance. We have had patients shot in the chest before with the bullet ripping through the heart muscle. Maybe it had torn one of the smaller upper chambers of the heart, the atriums. Hopefully, time and the paramedics' arrival were on the patient's side and then they would have a chance. It had to be quick to secure the airway with a tube, and to start the resuscitation immediately and get a blood pressure back. With an injury to the heart the surgeons may potentially crack the chest open, grab the rib spreader to flay the chest open, and jam a gloved finger into the gaping hole in the heart to stop the bleeding. That's if time was on your side.

Yes. We had done that too and cracked open other chests. The surgeon would jump on, and kneel on the stretcher beside the patient as she massaged the heart to keep it beating. She would have to get the blood to the rest of the body. We would make a mad dash down the hallways to the elevators to get to the operating room. A gunshot wound to the chest was often a deadly injury. A few made it, but most of them died. A success story was not going to be part of Lipson's workday today. Now, there was something else that he had to do, and he had to face the family. I saw the tears starting in Lipson's eyes.

"Now, I have to go tell this young man's family that their young son is dead," Lipson said. He shook his head in disbelief.

If he had continued his training in cardiac surgery, today he would probably have been putting in a catheter to unblock the hardened arteries in someone with heart disease. Or reading an ultrasound of the heart or interpreting a heart stress test report. He could have been involved in anything else today, but not this. Maybe his day would have been spent doing an angiography, an embolization, a microsurgery, but not this.

"Seven people shot," he said to himself again and stiffly marched away from me to go talk to the family. He was muttering quietly. I could not hear fully all what he was saying to himself. But, I am sure I clearly heard him say, "O, God, please, please, give me strength."

I had the cell phone to my ear, but had move the mouth piece away, and I don't think Bret could hear what Lipson was saying. Hopefully, he had not heard Lipson's conversation and think that I was talking to him. Lipson walked away to go into the family waiting room and lifted his head while he stood up straight. He pulled up both shoulders before stepping into the family room and gave the family the news.

I too silently shook my head and took a deep breath. I moved the phone's mouth piece back to my mouth and said:

"Bret, get me someone who will listen."

"The war is on. This is a war zone. We have to do something to stop the violence," I said.

"Unbelievable!" I said to no one in particular. Shooting a six year old at a parade. People were there to enjoy themselves, to celebrate an independence, an anniversary. It was to be a safe place with family and children. Shooting randomly into a crowd and shooting seven people, people who were simply trying to quietly live their lives and spend time with their families. It should have been safe.

"Bret, who do you know that we can talk to, Bret" I asked. "Bret, you know everyone."

"Please, Bret, please call now."

CHAPTER 15

A DAY FOR DECISION

"Hey, you guys, you can go over there," Carrie said, signaling with her head. She was trying to carry two trays at the same time, and take them to the kitchen that was at the back of the restaurant.

"Go to the table by the bay window." This time she spoke a little too loudly. The rest of the patrons looked up from their meals to see what the commotion was all about. Confident that nothing too dramatic was going to happen, they hunkered down to continue eating and talking to their dinner companions. All that drama was unnecessary. We knew what table she was talking about. We sat there all the time when we came to the Eatwell Diner. This diner was a favorite spot to hang out after work on Tuesdays.

We had just left a board meeting that had dragged on endlessly, and late into the evening. Lowell and I were on the board for the community organization. I liked being on the board. In addition to the community work that the organization was doing, I was also exposed to other people working in different industries who had different kinds of jobs. I had been on the board for only a year, but Lowell had been on it for more than five years. He knew about the past and present history of the organization. He knew all the historical data and could tell you why certain processes and people were in place today. Above all, he knew the people, what made them tick, what motivated them or not, how to push their buttons, and how to get under their skins.

"Yeah. You have to understand how and why it all happened. How it went down, you know. Then it will all make more sense to you," Lowell was fond of saying. He was a history major in college. Ask him any tidbit of information. I would think it was useless stuff. No, he knew it.

Of course, to understand the history of it all, that made sense. I knew that. If you knew the events in the past you were better able to interpret the events that you were seeing today. You may not understand it, but it may make more sense. You would have a better sense of people, their behaviors, and their motivations. Your interpretation of their actions or behaviors may not be perfect, but it adds a little bit of clarity to several pieces of the puzzle. At least you hoped it did.

It was a mystery why Lowell had not eaten all day. I tried to have a light breakfast every morning. Today though, my entire schedule seemed to be completely off kilter. I had been running late for everything and every meeting. My bio-clock was out of synch. It was not like I had pulled an all-nighter staying up or doing rotating shifts in the emergency room this week. But nonetheless, my circadian rhythm was completely off. Therefore, I was hopeful that I could use this time to unwind, eat a hearty meal, and get resynchronized. Carrie brought over two menus, and her assistant brought over two glasses of water.

"The usual drinks?" Carrie asked. I nodded yes, but Lowell said that he wanted to try something different. I started to look over the ample menu. The diner's menu had twelve pages. It was about four pages too long than any reasonable menu ought to. There was so wide a choice that you could easily become confused and lose focus on what you really wanted to eat. You could order from the breakfast, lunch or dinner menu anytime of the day. At midnight, patrons would be eating scrambled eggs and toast. This would really throw one's circadian rhythm off. The body would become confused, mistaking night for day and day for night. Eating this way created havoc on

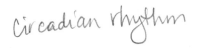

the mind and body. There was no structure, no defined pattern to guide the way. There was no consistency. Doing this jarred the mind and jerked the body around in its unpredictability.

Carrie handed us the menus so that we could look over the meal choices. However, she did not walk away from the table. She began to talk in haste and to ask questions. She started to talk very fast but, she always spoke in that manner. It was like listening to a run-on-thought spoken out in a run-on-sentence. You had to pay attention to get the gist of what she was saying. Where was she going with this line of questions? I tried to pick the sense out of the nonsense. When she told you about an event or why she opted not to do something, the rationale usually did not match with the root cause at hand. But, I was so used to her line of thinking that I peeled away the fluff and concentrated on the essence of the questions.

"Did you get the new television yet?" Carrie asked. She told us how she had gone to the casino and won two hundred dollars on the machine in the corner near the bright lights.

"You know, the one in the corner facing the man-made waterfalls," Carrie said. "You know the machine with flashing lights, and the loudest music possible this side of creation." Lowell nodded in agreement. He must have been very familiar with the casino, or he just nodded to be polite so that she would continue with her story. I had no clue what she was talking about so I just listened. I neither nodded in agreement nor shrugged to indicate cluelessness.

"So, G., did you get the new television set yet, or not?" Carrie asked. She called me G or G-man, I guess because to say my full name required too much effort after all that "chatter boxing" that she was doing. I shook my head to indicate, no, that I had not gotten the new television.

"So, what's up with that? What are you waiting for?" she asked.

"Well, for one, I want to wait for a great sale. For two, my current television works. And for three, I am not in any rush. I just saw those flat screen televisions and I wished I had one. But, it's not like I need one, you know what I mean?" I said.

"I want a new television, but I don't need one. But it just would be nice to move into the modern era," I said.

"Yeah, yeah. Trust me, he won't buy one, a flat screen TV, that is. He has already looked at three, if not four. He won't buy one, at least, not any time in this century."

"When he was buying his house, the realtor took him to, like thirty houses, and he bought the one that he saw from the third or fourth viewing," Lowell mocked.

"On many things he has good judgment and can make a decision. On other things it takes him forever to move off a dime," Lowell blurted out.

"Just like it is two different people. Split. Like Jack Nicholson in *One Flew Over the Cuckoo's Nest*, or Sally Field in *Sybil*. Split," Lowell said, bursting out and laughing uncontrollably.

"He has a personality flaw, I tell you," he said. "I have like known him forever and it took like two forevers for me to even find out that he has a brother. And he never wants to talk about him. A personality flaw I tell you."

"How's that even relevant?" I asked Lowell. I looked quizzically at Carrie.

"So what flat screen television do you suggest?" I asked Carrie so that we could change from my habits being the subject of the conversation. I had to listen intently to hear what she was saying. She spoke too fast with her lips moving quickly, and I had to strain to fully understand what she was saying.

"Oh, yeah. Get the newest and best brand. Go all the way. Splurge," Carrie said. I listened intently and watched her lips moving to decipher the information she was trying to give. I tried to read her lips without her seeing that I was doing this. I did not want her to think that I was staring.

"Oh yeah, I will buy that brand," I said. "Yeah, that one sounds like it's the best, and it won't break the bank," I said.

"Yeah. I can make a decision. I decided not to get one unless it was a super sale," I muttered to myself.

Carrie walked away to go to another table as the patrons were waving to get her attention. After she walked away, I returned to looking over the menu and saw that there was a Tuesday Special for princess chicken served over a bed of spaghetti. I could already savor the flavor of the juicy chicken smothered in tomato sauce and its spices. Lowell decided he would get the meatloaf. Just as we were about to wave Carrie over again to let her know that we were ready to place our order, she came back carrying cups of coffee for both of us. We always had coffee so she was correct in bringing it over as the second beverage.

"Hey, you guys came a little late tonight. More so than usual," she said.

"Yes. We got caught up in a meeting that dragged on and on. It went way over the time that was necessary to get through the agenda," I said.

"But I am starving, so give me the meatloaf," Lowell said.

"Yeah, and give me the Tuesday chicken special" I said.

"Are you kidding? Are you guys sure you want to have all that food so late at night?" Carrie asked. I looked up over my coffee mug. Good friends are good friends. But familiarity can breed contempt.

"Well, I am starving," I said.

"Yeah, I know," Carrie said, "but you guys came later tonight than your usual time."

"You know I mind my business. I don't step onto other people's turfs. I don't mean to interfere, but I am diabetic," Carrie said. "My doctor always tells me not to have such a heavy meal so late at night."

"I know I am a waitress and I should let you order whatever you want. But you guys are also my friends," Carrie said.

"You are going to eat that meal, and then you are going to go home, and not do anything else for the night. You are eating all those calories so late at night. And then the lack of physical activity so late in the day will only make you gain weight. That increased weight will increase your risk of becoming diabetic," Carrie said.

"Hey. I used to do the same thing," she added. "I did not do any physical activity. I did not go to the gym. I did not even walk around the block at home. I avoided all steps and anywhere there was an incline. I would park my car next to the closest entrance to get into any building. I would sit in my car near the building until a free space became available. I did not move at all. Then, I was munching on food all the time. I am around food all the time, so there was always the temptation to eat constantly. My mouth and stomach never got a period of rest," Carrie said.

"But, I went to the doctor and I found out I was diabetic. He told me to increase my physical activity and he made an appointment with a nutritionist, a registered dietitian. She went over my diet with me and she gave me suggestions of things to change in my diet."

"The small changes helped me to look at what I was eating and drinking. We did these changes to my meals and my eating so that I could lose weight. And, you know it was not a lot of weight to lose. The goal was to lose a small amount first and the effect on my diabetes was good. Just that small change in weight and it made such a difference."

"Of course, I also had to start taking medications for diabetes. I had to get my blood sugar under control. But, I feel much better now, and I do not feel so tired all the time. I have more energy now. Before this, I was feeling fatigued. I was eating all the time, was hungry all the time, and was peeing all the time," Carrie said.

"I did not feel well at all. I am glad that I went to the doctor. He told me what to do to get my blood sugar and diabetes under control," Carrie added.

"In fact, he told me he would work with me to watch my "ABCs." The "A" is for A1C. This is a blood test that he will get every three to six months to make sure that my blood sugar is under control. The "B" is for blood pressure. When you have diabetes, you have to have better control over your blood pressure. The doctor also told me he would put me on a blood pressure medication that would protect my kidneys from damage. The "C" is for cholesterol. Many diabetics also have high cholesterol. So my doctor checked my cholesterol level and put me on a medication to control my cholesterol. He gave me a team of providers, including the nutritionist, the pharmacist, and the foot and eye doctors to help me manage my diabetes."

"Carrie, you are so right," I said.

"Hey. Look at you. Tell me something that I don't know. Yep. I know I am right," Carrie said.

"Just because my doctor told me I have diabetes doesn't mean that I cannot do things to control my weight and my blood sugar."

"Physical activity is also good. So I plan to get moving with walking and doing some light sports. I like doing that anyway. I had just kept on telling myself that I didn't have the time. But, I needed to make the time."

"I am doing all this to reduce the risks of the complications from diabetes. I don't want any problems with my eyesight or kidney. I don't want heart problems or damage to the nerves in my body, hands, and feet."

"I don't want to be on dialysis. No, I am going to do everything to control my blood sugar. I don't want to be on a kidney machine."

"And, I don't want to have problems with circulation in my feet. I am going to do all that I can to reduce my risks for blood vessel problems. I want to not only prevent, but also to slow the risks of losing my toes, feet or legs. No, siree. I am going to take care of my body and my blood sugar," Carrie said.

Lowell was strongly shaking his head up and down in agreement with Carrie. "I am diabetic too," he said. "My doctor told me that too and I just did not listen to him then. Uhm. Know my "ABCs," huh? I like that and it's easy to remember," Lowell said.

"Lowell was diabetic?" He had not told me that, I said to myself. Well, I am glad that Carrie was always talkative and gave good advice.

"Carrie, you are so right. Let's see what else is on the menu that would be better at this time of night," I said. Carrie smiled.

"I know I am right. Look at page three, the healthy choices menu. I will give you a minute to look it over, and I will be back in a second to take your orders," she said. Lowell and I turned to the healthy choices menu, and looked over the meal choices that were there. We were certain to find something to eat that was healthier and better for this time of the night.

Waitress determined to ∆ & take care of her health.

I rapped on the door before walking into Room 10.

"Hey, Happy," Hope said to me and handed me the paper print out of the chart. Hope had seen me walking in the direction of the room with nothing in my hand. She assumed that I would need something to write notes on as I spoke to the patient. Hope was an excellent nurse and she was proactive and always gave good advice. She was an immigrant to the U.S. and had been here for over five years. She had been a nurse midwife in the island country where she was from. She was well educated, cheerful, and took pride in her work. She left her former life behind fleeing a bad marriage and abusive husband. She said that one day she would tell us her story how she came to Miami with only the clothes on her back, with no money, and only a determination to make a new life for herself far away from her husband.

"You are always so happy and you never seem to have a care in the world," Hope added.

I really did not need paper or a clipboard to record the story or history of what the patient would tell me. I knew the patient was Alexa. She had been to the emergency room many times before. All the emergency room staff knew her. We were like her primary care provider. It seemed that she did not like going to her primary care doctor for routine follow up. But then, her complaints usually meant that even if she called her doctor, and she gave her good advice and asked her to come to the office, Alexa would still come to the emergency room. I had now seen her three days in a row for chest pains. Today it was for another problem.

Uhm. Happy, uh? I asked myself. She always called me "Happy." That was the name she called me. Always seemed happy, uh? Can one really know what is going on in someone's mind? Everyone has a story to tell. We all walk around with our family history, the lives with our friends, the joys, the pains and scars of our lives hidden within us. You see our faces and our behaviors. But, is that enough so that you know what joys or scars one has? If I did not tell you my story, could you know it or know what I had been through?

Alexa was sitting up in the bed. She held the large plastic basin in front of her and had it placed on her lap. I walked around to the right side of the bed so that I could talk to her. The right side of the bed was the preferred side to complete the physical examination. If you failed to examine a patient from the right side of the bed when you were doing your clinical rotations in medical school, you'd better be sure that the instructor did not see you do that. That was a no-no and a reason for him or her to possibly give you a failing grade for that rotation.

Alexa started to vomit and she held her head over the pink plastic basin. She had not been fast enough when the vomiting started to get all the contents directed into the basin though. A wad of it landed on my shoes but I did not flinch. I grabbed two latex gloves from the box of gloves that was in the mounted holder on the wall. I then tore off a strip of cleaning wipes out of the plastic container that was sitting on the shelf. These containers were in every room to clean up before, during, and after each patient. I reached down and wiped the vomit from my shoes. I looked to see if there was any blood on them. There was none. I then tossed the wipes in the garbage container.

"Alexa, one second," I said, as I turned away to pull the gloves off, wash my hands, and dry them with the disposable paper towels. I signaled for

Hope to come into the room to take an order for a medication to stop the nausea and vomiting. I also looked in the basin. There was no blood in there either. I was glad that the vomiting was not projectile, for who knew where all that fluid would have ended up. I was used to the risk of exposure to all manner of body fluids. I made sure to cover up, used gloves, gowns, and eyewear protection, to minimize contact with my own skin. Sometimes though, the unexpected happen as was the case now.

Alexa had gastric bypass surgery last year as she had been overweight. She had become diabetic, had high blood pressure and high cholesterol levels. She was getting pain in her knees and hips. She told me that she had tried to lose weight all her life, but she had not been successful in doing so. She had been through several weight loss programs. She had been to a nutritionist. She would lose weight for a while, but had trouble keeping it off. She had gone to the gym and tried to be as physically active as her body allowed. Nothing seemed to help with her keeping the weight off. It was like being on a yo-yo with a string.

Eventually, her doctor referred her to a bariatric program, a program specializing in weight loss and weight loss surgery. Alexa had considered that all her options had been exhausted. She had all the testing done that the surgeon said was needed before he would consider doing surgery on her. She was seen by the cardiologist, the pulmonologist, and the psychologist. They asked her about alcohol and other substance use. They tested her for peptic ulcer disease and bacteria that are associated with stomach ulcers. She passed her tests with flying colors. She wanted to control her diabetes and her weight, and loved the thought of possibly not having to take all the medications that she had been taking. Though Alexa had passed all the pre-screening tests to have her gastric bypass surgery, she also suffered from panic attacks. She had been happy with the weight loss that she had achieved from the gastric bypass.

Anxiety disorders, which include panic disorder, generalized anxiety disorder, post-traumatic stress disorder, phobias, and separation anxiety disorder, are the most common types of mental disorders present in the general population. Today, I wanted to know why she was here. Was it a panic attack or a problem related to her gastric bypass? Was she here because she had overeaten or was she here due to a possible complication from the gastric bypass surgery? I decided to start over to understand what the problems were today.

"Good morning, Alexa. I see that you are vomiting," I said. It was great that she had lost weight and had gotten her diabetes under control using this surgery, even if this method was not for everyone.

"What brings you to the emergency room today?" I asked, very curious to understand why she was in the emergency department this time.

In the ICU

"Dr. Gary," Dana said. "We need you to come to the Burn Unit."

"What for?" I asked.

"One of the patients has extubated himself," Dana said. Why had the patient chosen to pull out the tube that hooked him to the ventilator, the breathing machine? How was he going to breathe? Was he confused, demented, agitated, or in pain? Or had he just given up on life? Was he depressed, dejected, feeling helpless and hopeless?

"Uhm. We need the tube back in," she said.

"Can you come now to replace the tube?" Dana asked.

"Sure. Sure. I will be right there," I said.

"Could you please have the intubation tray and the necessary medications ready and at the bedside for me?" I asked.

"Hey. I am way ahead of you. You don't even have to ask. Being prepared? You know I would do that, right?" Dana replied.

"I will have the tray and the meds at the bedside. You take a seven and a half glove, right? Do you want the latex gloves or the nitrile gloves?" she asked.

"No. Latex is fine. I don't have a latex allergy, at least not yet. No, I take eight gloves," I said. Sometimes the eight fit too closely and my fingers felt constricted in the gloves that I could not maneuver the laryngoscope and detachable blades. A laryngoscope was the small metal equipment that we used to see the epiglottis and vocal cords. I preferred to use the curved blade for guidance, lifting the soft tissues of the neck so that I could see the vocal cords to put the airway tube in. Some other doctors preferred the straight blade to do this procedure, but this was really a matter of personal preference for the most part.

Dana was always well prepared. So I was sure that she would have both types of blades and in different sizes, just in case one was needed. I arrived in the Burn Unit less than two minutes later.

"What's up?" I asked Dana.

"Oh, he pulled the ventilator tube out by himself," she replied.

"We had lightened his sedation somewhat. His hands were free and he pulled the tube out," she replied.

"Well, obviously, he can breathe on his own," I said.

"Well yes, he can, but he really needs to be sedated and given more pain medications," she said.

"He was burned over fifty percent of his body," she said.

"It is late at night, we don't want him to be off the vent overnight," she said.

"Besides, he needs sedation and more pain meds. We need to protect his airway and breathing. Everything is at the bedside."

I looked over the chart and history, the medications and notes on the prior intubation. There were no allergies, and there were no complications or problems when he was first intubated. We walked to the bedside. She and I both put gloves and masks on and started the procedure to place the airway tube back in. It turned out to be a fairly straightforward procedure. The man had a long thin neck, and after the sedation was given, the muscles around his neck relaxed enough to place the tube into the airway. The respiratory tech took over at that point. We confirmed the placement of the tube by the various procedures and the tech placed him back on the vent.

"Wow, that's too bad that he got burned like that," I said.

"Yes," Dana said. "What I heard is that he had a meth lab in his apartment. I don't know what he was doing, but there was an explosion and he got severely burned. He is fortunate to have survived the explosion. I only hope the authorities can root out more of these illegal meth labs and prevent these kids from getting hurt, either by the drug itself, or from explosions like these. That's a terrible burn," she said.

"I know, I know," I said.

"We need to really look at the drug and substance abuse issue and come up with a plan to prevent and to eliminate it."

"Yes. We should do something about this as it's a growing problem," Dana said.

I like this survey of
other systemic issues:
gun violence
diabetes/obesity
addiction/drugs (meth lab)
anxiety
The thread of history - how do we
understand a problem?

CHAPTER 16

PAIN BUT NO GAIN

S arah had the foresight to put on a mask before coming with me into the exam room. She had done her assessment and had known what to expect. She had offered me a mask too.

"You will need this," she said. I had hesitated and had not put the mask on before going into the room. That was a mistake. Immediately, I was struck by a sweet pungent smell that slammed into my nostrils and assaulted my brain. What smell was that? My brain was trying to figure out if it had smelled anything like that before. It tried to decode the type of odor and it was completely confusing. It jarred a memory but I could not pinpoint the mixtures of that foul smell. Sarah stood to the left of the bed and I stood to the right.

"Hi, Ms. Morris, I am Dr. Gary," I said. "How are you?"

"Do you mind if I put my mask on?" I asked. Ms. Morris shook her head indicating that she did not mind.

"Can I have one too?" she asked.

"Absolutely," Sarah said and pulled a mask out of the box on the wall.

"I understand that you have a lump on your breast," I said.

"Yes," Ms. Morris responded.

"How long has it been there?" I asked.

"Oh, a while," she said.

"Oh, what's a while?" I asked.

"Well, I have had it for more than a year, but it started to get bigger over the last month," she said.

"Do you mind if we take a look while I ask you some more questions?"

"Not at all," she replied. Ms. Morris gingerly pulled away the gown to uncover her right breast. Sarah and I did not react to what we saw, but I had to take a deep breath. The source of the odor was now obvious. There was a large fungating mass that took up half of the right breast. The skin of the breast was classic *peau d'orange*. It looked like the skin of an orange, was thickened, swollen, stippled with dimpling from the mass and the irritation that lay within it. The nipple was pulled in, and there was an open draining area immediately north of the nipple that oozed a bloody substance mixed with pus. This was more than an abscess; this was a cancer of the breast.

"You have only had this for a year?" I asked, slightly pulling down my mask so that my voice would not be muffled.

"Well, I had noticed a lump for a while."

"It got bigger and became painful. The skin opened and it started draining over the last week or two," she added.

"Do you have a doctor?" I asked.

"No."

"When was the last time that you saw a doctor?"

"A while."

I guessed that a while meant years, but at least one year. Had she not had any preventive care? Even if she had no insurance, did she know that there are community clinics in the city where she could get health care for free or pay only a small fee? There were also programs run by the city health department and hospitals that provided free mammograms to women who had no insurance. Was she aware of that? Even if that were the case, that she did not know that programs existed and were available to do free screenings and mammograms, wasn't that mass and breast irritation extremely painful?

Was there something else that prevented her from going to the doctor or hospital? If pain alone did not force her to come for help, did something else prevent her from coming?

Aside from non-melanoma skin cancer, breast cancer is the most common cancer among women in the United States. It is also one of the leading causes of cancer death among women of all races. Different people have different warning signs for breast cancer. Some people do not have any signs or symptoms at all. A person may find out they have breast cancer after a routine mammogram.

Some of the warning signs of breast cancer are a new lump in the breast or armpit; thickening or swelling of part of the breast; irritation or dimpling of breast skin; redness or flaky skin in the nipple area or the breast; pulling in of the nipple or pain in the nipple area; nipple discharge other than breast milk, including blood; any change in the size or the shape of the breast and pain in any area of the breast. Keep in mind that some of these warning signs can happen with other conditions that are not cancer.

"Ms. Morris, have you ever had a mammogram?" I asked.

"What is a mammogram?" she asked.

I wanted to make sure that I explained it in terms that she would understand.

I needed to speak to make sure that I would not confuse her. Besides, I would also have to give her the news that she would not be going home tonight. I intended to call the surgeons to get her admitted to the hospital. She would need some work on the breast mass. I would need to do more tests. She would probably end up in the operating room tonight and while doing surgery, the surgeons would take a sample and send it to the pathologist to tell us if it was cancer and what type.

"A mammogram is an X-Ray picture of the breast," I said.

"We use this picture to look for early signs of breast cancer."

"Why should I get a mammogram?" Ms. Morris asked.

"Well, having a regular mammogram is the best test for doctors to find breast cancer early. We doctors can also show you how to feel for lumps in your breast. But sometimes it takes up to three years before you feel a lump," I said.

"So, a mammogram is better to look for breast cancer even before you can feel a lump. When we can find the breast cancer early, many women go on to live long and healthy lives," I said.

"Well, I already knew something was wrong," she said.

"But, I was so afraid. I did not want to know what I had, and I did not want to come to the doctor. But the pain and smell got to be too much and I had to come," she said.

"I know, I know," I said, looking over at Sarah, who looked sad. I thought that even if we had not gotten the prevention message to Ms. Morris, maybe she would tell her friends and family to talk to their health care provider about getting a mammogram.

"Ms. Morris, tell your family and friends to talk to their health care provider if they have any symptoms or changes in their breast. Tell them to let their health care provider know if someone in their family has breast cancer. The health care provider will let them know how often they should get a mammogram based on their age and their family history. There are guidelines to follow about that."

"Do you have any questions for me or Sarah?" I asked.

"No," Ms. Morris said. "I already know it is cancer. My mother had breast cancer. Her mother and my aunts had it as well. I just didn't want to know, I just wanted it to go away but I had to come after the pain started," she said.

"I already have depression so I did not want to cope with bad news."

"Well, I am glad you did not wait any longer and came today," I said.

"This way we can do something about this problem, and also let you talk to someone about your depression, if you would like," I said.

"We will need to keep you in the hospital tonight and I will call some other doctors too to help you. They may have other tests they want you to have," I said.

"Once they take a piece of the lump, they can give you advice about what to do next. Does, that sound okay?" I asked. "Sarah will stay with you a bit," I said.

She nodded yes and started to cry. I quietly turned and walked out of the room to call the surgeons. Sarah stayed with her to answer any questions, to tell her about the admission process, and to let her know about a peer support group that the hospital had for patients with breast cancer.

A Head Injury

Sam sat on the chair while I stood behind him and draped the towel around his shoulders. I was getting ready to cut his hair as I did his weekly grooming. First, I would cut his hair then I would shave him. If he could sit still after all that activity I would then trim his finger nails. I had to plan and work quietly and quickly because for the most part, he would not sit still long enough to do all three activities.

"Don't cut my hair too low this time," Sam said.

"You always cut it too low," Sam insisted. "I don't want my hair as low as you keep yours." I tended to keep my hair on the low side, as I thought it looked better that way and it was simple.

"Okay, I won't take too much hair off." I repositioned the towel to cover the back of Sam's neck. I chose the number three hair guide, placed it on the hair trimmer, and turned the trimmer on. Sam looked up and flinched when he heard the quiet buzzing of the blades going back and forth. I placed the trimmer against his scalp going from the left side to right side in a constant pattern. I moved next to the crown to trim the hair into an even hairstyle. I still thought the length of the hair was too long, so I replaced the number three guide with a number two hair guide and repeated the motions.

"Don't take too much off," Sam said again.

"I am not," I said to reassure him. I trimmed down the sides and then turned attention to the middle again. I moved the trimmer from the top of his head near the forehead and worked the trimmer backwards to the nape of the neck. Sam was right. I had taken too much of the hair off at the crown. Now, with the thinning hair at the middle worked down by the number two hair guide, the jagged four-inch healed gash was visible. The scar left a ridged mountain that had been hidden by the height of his hair. Now my insistence to get his hair a little lower and neater had exposed the jagged gash in his scalp for everyone in the world to see. It was obvious if you stood or sat behind him, and the only way to hide it now was to wear a hat.

I tried to ignore my mistake and continued to trim to get all the sides even. As the buzzing trimmer went closer to Sam's scalp again he nervously flinched. I had seen the head injury before and I saw it every week when I cut his hair. Was he having any symptoms of PTSD – post traumatic stress disorder symptoms – related to this injury? I wondered about the persons who had traumatic brain injuries and how it affected their lives.

I remembered the night when the paramedics called for help with a situation. They were on the scene with an accident and they were not sure if they should bring the person in or not.

I stood over Sam and a wave of nausea came over me. I felt lightheaded.

That night the red emergency phone seemed to ring more loudly than ever before. Sylvie, the paramedic who had answered the call, was on scene with the others. I knew the raspy southern drawl of her voice and she was now speaking in a rapid sequence. Her words were very clear, crisp, calm, but forceful. One could recognize her voice anywhere even in a room with everyone loudly talking. She did not have to speak loudly for you to distinguish the sound of her voice from the others. It was just so distinctive in tone and quality that it was recognizable after her just saying one or two words.

The charge nurse answered the emergency phone.

"This is EMT Unit 4," Sylvie said.

"We are on scene with a male who jumped off a three story building," she continued.

"We need Med Control," Sylvie said.

"We need Med Control, please," Sylvie repeated.

Lena, the charge nurse who had answered the phone, waved to me as I peered out of the fishbowl. The fishbowl was the glass enclosed area where the doctors sat and completed their charting in the medical record. Lena wiggled her index finger to tell me to come to the phone to provide Med Control to Unit 4. I quickly got up and went over to the nursing station where Lena was standing.

"They need Med Control," Lena whispered, cradling the phone between her left ear and shoulder and covering the phone's mouth piece with her hand. She was quickly scribbling, with her right hand, pieces of information on a scrap of paper.

"What's wrong?" I asked.

"I don't know yet," Lena said, shrugging her shoulders.

"Hi. This is Dr. Gary, Med Control number 123."

"What do you have?"

"This is Unit 4. We are on scene with a man who jumped off a building. He hit his head on landing. His skull is open and you-know-what is coming out."

Not again I pleaded.

"Did you get the vitals? Is he breathing still? Is there a blood pressure and heart rate?"

"Yes. We did. He was barely breathing. We secured his neck and put a tube in his airway. He still has a blood pressure and a heartbeat."

"Well, don't call it on the scene," I said.

"Is that your question? To call it on scene and pronounce him dead on scene?"

"Yes," Sylvie said.

"Christ. You really can't, not like that," I said. "Bring him in and do all the medications as you normally would. Let's see what we have when you get here. Don't call it on scene. Get out of there and bring him in."

I steadied my hand on the last track of hair on Sam's scalp. I had seen too many of those suicides and attempted suicides in the emergency room. Was there a way for us to reach these young men and women before they went from helplessness to hopelessness? What did we have to do to stop it? I hoped and prayed to find a way.

TIP BOX 4

1. Life has ups and downs: Anchor yourself in a source of strength to make it through the hard times

2. No one wants to come onto a sinking ship: Do not take on commitments that you cannot fulfill. Be comfortable with saying, "NO"

3. Remember to rest and relax: This is essential for you to rejuvenate your mind and body

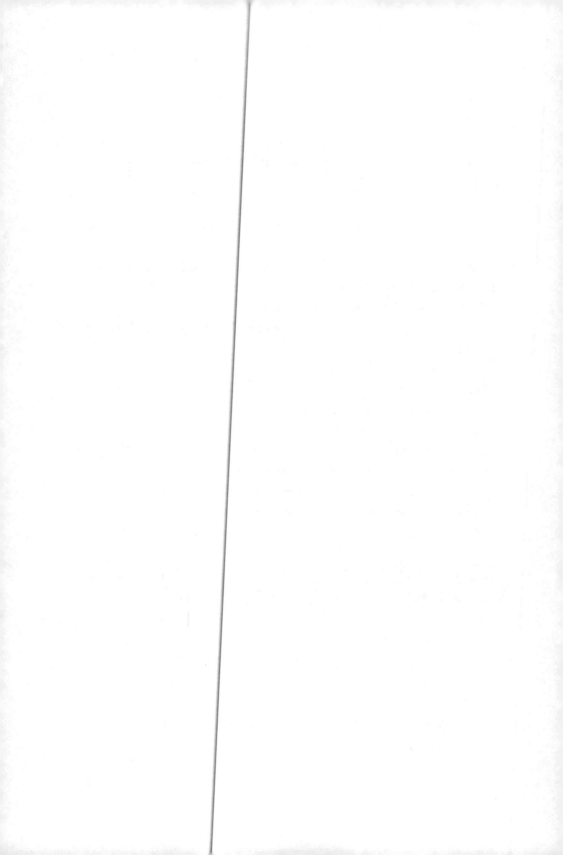

PART V

DAYS OF RAIN

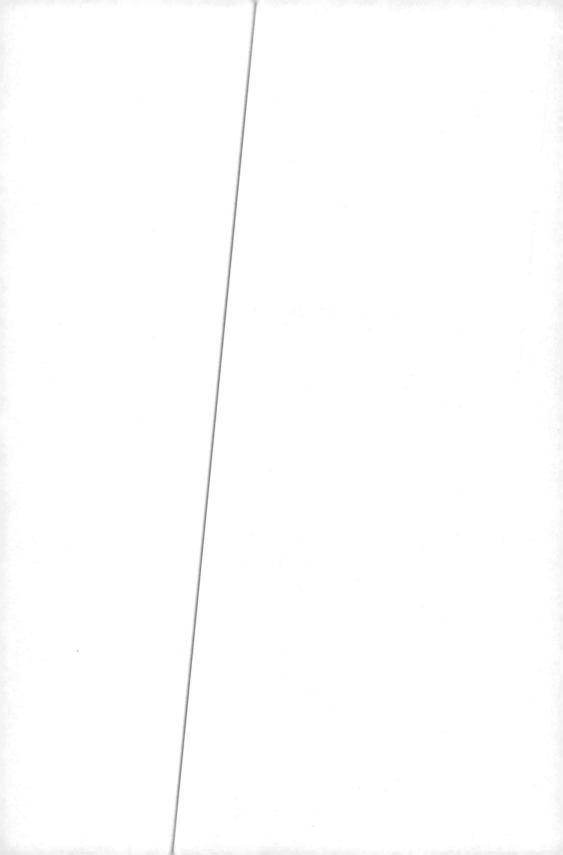

Double Negative

No,
Not never.
You can't ever do that
Dream…
A future with peace,
Dumb fool—
No one, not never,
Could ever do that.
Dream…
Will never, not
Be that,
Silly idiot—
Sit down and shut up,
Don't think,
Don't move,
Don't dream,
Don't speak, not never,
Dream…
Your motive?
Hate?
The ugliness in me to create?
Brain in schism,
Born to negate,
Can't relate.
You motivate me,
Dream…
To be double negative,
Dream…

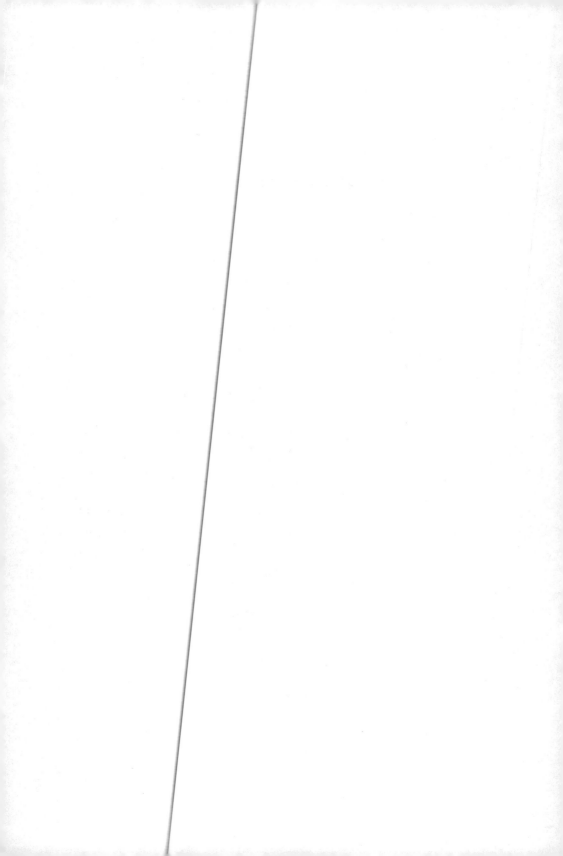

CHAPTER 17

DIZZY DALLIANCE

Lucea was fond of saying that fish rot at the head. She said that in fact it first became obvious in the eyes.

"Look at the eyes and see how dull, glassy, and lifeless they are," she said.

"When the fish's eyes lose that vibrant color and are cloudy, the fish had been dead before it had been removed from the water by the fisherman. Even if the body looked like it was full of life, the fish was dead. This is similar to people."

"We first die in the mind and soon thereafter the body goes as well. Heal the mind, heal the body."

Lucea was my cousin. I was glad that she volunteered to stay at my house with Sam and Esther while I was away for the week on a medical mission. Lucea looked at my eyes and said, "It looks like you need a break."

"You know, the caretaker has to take care of himself first. If you do not, you cannot take care of anyone else. Your eyes look lifeless and you really need to take a vacation."

It was always good to listen to good advice. Dr. Hunter, who had coordinated this medical mission had also called and warned me not to cancel this time. On the last planned trip to Belize I had to bail at the last minute as I had no one to help me with Sam. I could not just get up and go one thousand miles away and have no way of getting back home quickly. Besides, I was not even sure what kind of technology would be available there. Would my cell phone work there? Could I even log on to the internet to send an email? I really had not done my homework to be sure that I would not be disconnected from the rest of the world in case of an emergency. Though I knew the team was disappointed that I had canceled at the last minute, I felt that it was the best decision given all my options. Still, Dr. Hunter didn't let me off the hook that easily.

"The last time you said you would come with us you cancelled. I know that you have other obligations at home and that you take care of your brother. But sometimes you need a respite from all of that. You need to find

out what recharges your batteries and just do it. Because if you do not do that you won't have enough energy to run this marathon called life."

"Hey. This is not a sprint. I take care of my elderly father at home as well and he is in poor health. You have to pace yourself and ask for help. If you don't, you won't be able to finish the race. You have to take care of yourself first. If you do not, you cannot take care of anyone else."

But, in fact, this was not a vacation. I went there to work. But, I liked to volunteer for medical missions in other countries. It was good to experience another culture and to understand different perspectives on life and medicine.

The flight down to Jamaica was slightly more than three hours from New York. It was nice to be going back to my native land after not visiting there for a long time. It was also a while that I had done any medical voluntary work in Jamaica. We landed in Kingston and then drove the rest of the way to Port Antonio, Portland. I was starting to relax and getting used to the surroundings when on the second day we had a cultural immersion. We had finished our work day and on our way back to the apartments where we were staying.

We were chatting and looking out the car window when a rickety bicycle whizzed by the line of cars that was cautiously going down the curved road of the hillside. There was no way the rider could see beyond the sharp upcoming curve in the road. The rider sped himself and his bicycle headlong on the right side of the road, and he was going straight into the oncoming traffic from the opposite side.

"What? Did you see that? Did you see the guy on the bicycle?" I asked Vivian, the dentist, who had joined the volunteer team on the mission trip.

Vivian looked at the bicycle rider, and rolled her eyeballs into her head to express disbelief at what she was seeing.

"Of course, I saw it," she said.

"What was that?"

I grinned trying to hide the fear and discomfort of seeing what was like an accident just waiting to happen. The risks that people take when on the road, whether in a car, truck, or bicycle, were alarming. I don't think that I always thought about the risks that they took until I started to work in the emergency room, and I saw the end product of the injuries to life and limb.

Even though I grew up in Kingston, I left before learning to drive on this side of the road. I refused to drive here as the island's drivers drove their cars on the left side of the roadway. I became too confused trying to figure out on what side of the road I should be. Whenever I got to the roundabouts, which were numerous on the island's road, I could not determine who had the right of way in the circle. I preferred today to sit in the back seat and look out of the window enjoying the scenery. I sat in the rear passenger's seat and that meant that going down this hill, to my immediate left was a sheer precipice into a green nothingness.

"Huh," I thought to myself, "there are no barriers between the roadway and the drop off. Where is the Jersey barrier, or steel guided border, or preferably a solid concrete retainer wall? Did they just not get to building it yet?"

Clarence, the local taxi driver who the volunteer group had asked to drive us around the island today, barely looked at the bicycle rider. He was as calm and cool as ever. He was not nervous probably from the years of experience driving these same roads. Clarence seemed to know every nook, cranny, and where all the potholes were in the road. He nimbly avoided all of them, large or small. It did not matter if they suddenly appeared in the roadway or not.

I had taken a good look at the body of the car to see if the threads on the tire were worn down before I had gotten into the car. I also watched Clarence to see if his hands were shaking, or if he seemed physically weak. I chatted him up asking him so many questions that he got tired of me asking them. I was only trying to figure out if he was drunk. Did his judgment appear intact? If he were to drive me and the team along these insanely curvy roads, would I feel comfortable or would I have palpitations in the back seat?

This part of the island was beautiful as there was greenery everywhere. It was unlike Kingston, the fast paced city, which had people, buildings, cars, and jammed-packed buses everywhere. This area was a tropical rainforest and the trees were tall, lush, and sturdy. The leaves had made good use of the sun in its photosynthesis. Every tree had a fruit of some sort or another. The shrubbery was thick and colorful and there was water everywhere. Should there really be any hungry child or person here? Should we not be able to harvest the bounty of the land and use what the earth had generously provided?

We were working at Port Antonio Hospital in the heart of the city. However, the hospital was perched on the top of a small hill. The road to get up there had a sharp incline and without good lungs or good legs, by the time you got to the top you were breathless. The view from there was spectacular. The first day was clear so we could see far away into the distant sea and see a small island called Navy Island. No wonder Errol Flynn and his cronies had come to this part of the world for rest and relaxation. The air was fresh and clean and the sun light permeated your body with its natural healing qualities. The hospital was first opened as a tuberculosis sanatorium, and that was why it was situated away from street level and the people. The thought was that the fresh air would cleanse the lungs, and the constant view of the clear aqua bluish-green sea would touch the mind and heal the body.

Nowadays, though, having the hospital clinging off the side of a hill was not such a good idea. If you were sick and on foot, the climb up would be treacherous, and you would need resuscitation once you got to the hospital's front steps. If you made it up there on foot, it would have been only by sheer willpower. That is why the kindness of strangers was welcomed as you bummed a ride in a car, or were forced to pay a taxi to get up there when you were at your most feeble and most in need. Either way, once I saw the breathtakingly beautiful view I fell in love again with the island.

The bicycle rider must have reached his destination. As we continued to slowly proceed down the hillside, I looked to the left and to right to make sure he was not sprawled in the roadway. Vivian and everyone were looking intently now as well. Alternately, we looked at the scenery.

Vivian pointed upward.

"Wow, look at that!" she exclaimed.

"Look at that house just suspended there like that."

We glanced to the right and upward to look at a house serenely perched at the edge of the hill. The tangerine colored house dangled too dangerously close to the edge. It was perched on concrete stilts anchored to a solid foundation in the rocks. The hospital had been built on a hill too so being able to look up and look out was admired here.

"Wow. Wow," I said. Everything and everybody needs a source of anchoring. When Sam was lurching at the edge of insanity, isn't that what he tried to do? To find a thread of life on which to cling? Is that tangerine house any different from anything else in life that we try to do?

All of us stared at the house and the magnificence all around us. Only the driver seemed indifferent to it. We glanced at the roadway and silently prayed: "Let's not see the bicyclist lying in the roadway at the next corner, please, God, please."

During our time in Port Antonio the medical team treated over two hundred patients. We took blood pressures and did physical examinations. We gave them information about high blood pressure, diabetes, good hygiene, sanitation, and drinking clean water. We talked about physical activity to help prevent long term medical problems. We gave them toothbrushes, bandages, eyeglasses, and gloves. The dental team pulled a few rotten teeth. We promised the next time to partner with the local health providers to help with treatment and follow up care for the work that we did and the problems that we saw.

I did not know how common mental illness was here, and we did not bring a mental health provider on our team. I assumed that like most places they had their share of depression, schizophrenia, post-traumatic stress disorder, panic, anxiety, and bipolar disorders. I also thought they would

medical mission

have the entire spectrum of childhood and adult injuries, domestic violence, maltreatment, and violence. I took a mental note to find out more about this the next time I was here. Everywhere we went people kept on saying, "No problem, mon." Maybe that was their mantra to free their minds, to calm their nerves, and to enjoy their lives.

With the people here walking up those steep hills to their homes, physical inactivity was probably not one of their problems, at least not in this part of the island.

"We call that 'dallying,'" Clarence said, breaking the silence and now speaking.

"The bicycle rider, he can dally," Clarence repeated.

It was a dizzying dalliance and I closed my eyes to block the memory of it.

I just did not want to think about the young woman who had lost her legs after she was hit by the train. My chest ached when I imagined how Sam was clinging and fighting for his own sanity without help being there. Clinging, perching, dangling on a too thin thread barely anchoring him on the positive side of reality.

I did not want to repeat the experiences of any traumas. Not here in Port Antonio. Not now. Not ever.

Leaf of Life

I was happily looking forward to a day of rest that was scheduled after our volunteer work in Port Antonio had ended. The day of relaxation was the day before we were to leave. The volunteers voted, and we all agreed to spend the last day rafting on the Rio Grande. None of us had gone rafting before and so it seemed like a good idea. It would be a different experience from the usual lying on the beach and basking in the sun. The tour guide told us that rafting on a bamboo raft would be something that we would never forget. He insisted that the boost would energize us to go on to the next phases of our lives when we returned home.

A day of rest was welcomed after seeing so many patients over the last week. We saw patients with thyroid goiters as big as oranges. I also never thought I would ever see a patient who had a hernia as large as a basketball walking around not bothered by it. I was taking his blood pressure and I noticed it as he sat there.

"How long have you had that hernia?" I asked.

"Oh. You mean 'the growth'?" he asked.

"Oh, for a while. I have had this for a while."

He has had that hernia for many years. I guessed that the reason that he had not done anything about it before was that he could not pay a doctor. After this long time, the hole in his groin would have gotten bigger. Now, most likely more than half of his gut lay in it. He did not want anyone to look at it.

"Oh, no, I don't want them to cut me," he said triumphantly. "It is not bothering me so, I am not bothering it," he said.

He shrugged his shoulders as I was trying to explain the seriousness of his condition. I was saying that sometimes the gut gets trapped and cannot go back into the upper belly. That's where it belonged. If the gut got trapped in the hernia, we say the hernia is incarcerated, and that means it is jailed or locked up. He shrugged again as I continued to explain.

"You know, the gut can also get blocked and that's a real emergency," I said.

"Or if the gut gets trapped and enough blood does not get to it, it would get strangled. Where are you going to go if that happened?" I asked.

He stood his ground and was not having any of it. He was done. He was not going to take care of it at all. That was it and he did not want anyone to cut it.

"No, I have had it for a long time. I don't want it touched. Never. They will never cut me," he said decisively. "Never, not now. Ever." *hernia*

"Let things be as they are. I can deal with whatever happens," he said.

"I have lived a long and good life. I can deal with whatever happens," he said.

I nodded.

"Why even press the point?" I asked myself.

In any case, we did not have a surgeon with us and could not do anything for him now anyway. Maybe if he had the money he would go into the town to see one of the doctors there. But, it was obvious he had no intention of doing even that. He was living quite happily with the large hernia, and no amount of information or cajoling would make him change his mind.

I accepted his resolve and his right to make his own choice. I continued working and took his blood pressure and listened to his heart. These were both fine.

"Is my blood pressure good?" he asked.

"Oh. Yes. It is perfect," I replied.

He then told me how he kept his blood pressure down with chewing garlic daily and by walking everywhere he went.

"You know, I either chew some garlic or I make a tea with it," he said. "Yes, sir. Garlic is good for a lot of things. Whenever I have a cough, I make a tea of garlic and put in a small amount of olive oil. I take one teaspoon of the mixture in the morning, and one teaspoon in the evening. In no time, my cough is gone," he said.

"You know what, Doc? I also use a sorrel drink that is good for blood pressure, or to lower my cholesterol," he said. "Oh, you know sorrel as hibiscus," he said.

"Doc?" he asked.

"You know what? You should come back to Port Antonio. Next time I will tell you all about the spices and herbs that we have in our little island paradise. God has given us all that we need to live and be happy, right here on this piece of rock," he said.

"Yes. Yes. Of course, I will come back," I promised.

I shook his hand and thanked him for all the advice. I also made a mental check to return for him to tell me and the other volunteers about the herbs, spices, and leaves, and the many uses to heal the body and the mind.

Three Girls in Blue

The old rickety taxi constantly belched and sputtered going up the steep hill to get to the starting point of the rafting station.

At the starting point we were assigned a guide to take the team down the Rio Grande. The starting station was a sparsely furnished one-room building. It was said to be the office, and its location was ideal as it was at a broad and level area near the river bank. This was a wide pool area where the river had slowed to a standstill. Our guide was well tanned as his head was perpetually exposed to the sun, wind, and rain. He did not wear a cap or any other cover on his head. He appeared to be in his forties and he was thinly built. All the muscles of his arms, the triceps and biceps, bulged and were very well developed. His legs were more than sturdy. Like his head, his feet were not covered. His heels were calloused and his soles were as cast iron to protect his bare feet. His toenails were starting to curl at the toes' edge and needed cutting.

He walked up to us and smiled broadly. All his teeth were white except some of the incisors were missing, and a few other teeth were jagged and in disrepair.

"Good morning, I am Colin. Colin Treadwell is my name," he said.

"But, you may call me "Teddy" though; all my friends call me that."

Teddy made sure he talked to everyone in the group and he had an easy smile for each. He looked happy that he had greeted us all individually. We exchanged the usual pleasantries that were required at this time of morning and he smiled at each of us again and asked "Ready?"

He was telling us that it was time to start the rafting, and he walked excitedly with us down to the mooring of the bamboo rafts.

He smiled again and sized each of us, looking us up and down. When he had completed his assessment, he broke the team apart and put us in pairs.

"You have to go with her. And you with him," he said to different pairs. "You have to go like this so that the raft will have the proper balance," he said. "Here are the other guides for the rest of you," he added.

"You have to balance," he said.

"If not, going down the river is harder. You need balance. If you are not balanced in the water, you will find yourself in the water."

He looked like he knew what he was doing; we nodded and paired up to get into the bamboo rafts. I sat beside Vivian, the dentist. Teddy nimbly hopped to the front of the bamboo raft. He used a long sturdy bamboo shaft as a lever to push us away from the bank of the river and the raft immediately glided from the edge of the river bank.

Teddy steered the raft to the center of the river where the water's flow was constant. He tested the river's depth there with the bamboo stick, and he struck the bottom of the river bed with it to get a sense of its depth. Then, in one fluid motion, he pushed off the river bed to propel the raft forward.

The river's flow helped with the forward motion of the raft. Now that we settled in an easy motion, Teddy had time to talk. Teddy began by repeating his name.

"Yes, I am Colin Treadwell, but everyone calls me Teddy. I love the river."

The raft bobbed and weaved on the water, but it was steady and balanced. He stood at the narrow section at the front of the raft, and Vivian and I were closer to the back sitting on an elevated seat. The seat was also made of bamboo and held together by a coarse rope. The seats had a backrest on which you could lean back on. Teddy had also outfitted the seats with soft cushions. Comfort was important for the ride Teddy explained, as we would be sitting on the raft for about three hours, the duration of the trip down this strip of the river.

The river flowed quietly but rapidly. At this part of the river Teddy did not have to do a lot of rowing or pushing with the bamboo stick. Yet, he held the bamboo firmly in his hand. He was prepared for anything. He stood there strongly and firmly. Though he appeared relaxed, you knew he was watching and well prepared for any change in the river. He rested sinewy arms on the bamboo and chatted away to keep us entertained.

"Oh, look into the water. There are some mullets and jangas," he said. "Those are fish that love this part of the river. The water is cooler in that section and there is plenty of food for them here."

"You know, I am seventy years old," he started again.

The bamboo raft meandered quietly down the Rio Grande, and I looked at him in surprise. Vivian and I looked at each other. It must be in the water. How was that possible? Everyone appeared to be younger than the age they told us they were. What were they doing that was so different from what I was doing?

Vivian and I looked at arms and a body structure that was well developed, but not bulky. You could tell that he had remained fit by doing physical activity all his life. His work helped with that as this was hard work repeatedly rowing down this river.

Well, obviously, some of it had to do with genetics. There was something about his family history that allowed him to age at a slower pace than others. It must be a complex interplay of genetics, the environment, and what he

in Jamaica

was eating daily. This was the usual nature versus nurture debate. "How long have you been doing this work?" Vivian asked.

"Oh. More than fifty five years," he said. We almost fell out of our seats to pitch out of the raft. What? What? Working that long in this sun and rowing daily? How did he do it? Just when we were about to ask him more questions, Teddy deftly grabbed the bamboo stick. He slowed the bamboo raft to almost a standstill. Immediately ahead of us, Teddy looked at three girls in blue crossing the river at a shallow part of the river. The girls smiled and waved at Teddy and us.

"Why are they in the river?" I asked.

"They are going home," Teddy said.

"Home? Here? Here in the river?" I asked.

Teddy pointed the bamboo shaft towards the beach and upwards towards a small hill facing the river.

"They live there," he said, still pointing up the small hill.

"They go to the primary school in the town and they walk to school. When school is over they walk back home," Teddy said.

"See. Their uniforms are blue and they wear white shirts," he said. "There's only one school, anyway. But, you know where they go to school," he added.

I watched in amazement as the three girls in blue crossed the river. They held their shoes in one hand, and in the other hand they held their school books. None of them had a backpack.

Teddy waved happily again at the girls as they reached the other side of the river. The hems of the blue uniforms were wet from the crossing, and they dropped their shoes on the sandy beach to put them back on while waving goodbye.

We spent another hour coming down the river and by then it felt like home as Teddy told us everything about the river. He knew the names of all the trees, flowers, and shrubs. He stared at the water and named all the different fish, snails, and shrimp.

Too soon the rafting came to an end. I could first hear the lap, lap, lapping of the waves as the river joined with the open sea, and the lapping became louder as we entered the mouth of the sea. At a point just before the raft would go under a bridge across the river, Teddy steered the raft to a small landing that had four stone steps. He steadied the raft and jumped to the bank. Once it was tied to a mooring, he helped us get out of the bamboo raft.

"Wow!" Vivian and I both said. "That was three hours in this lifetime that was well spent."

Rafting on the Rio Grande was a restful and peaceful experience. The tour guide was correct in recommending this activity over others that the team could have done. I was now ready to go back home and face any task. It did not matter how challenging or daunting it would be.

If the girls in blue could cross a wide river and still wave and smile, what was there in life that could not be conquered and overcome? I counted my blessings and put all the things in my life that I was complaining about in perspective and breathed to enjoy the rafting and river's journey.

CHAPTER 18

RESUSCITATED

I teleported my entire body through the telephone lines. I was speaking into the telephone, but I felt that there was a disconnect between the words that I was speaking and what by brain was thinking. I was convinced that what I was saying and what my brain was trying to make me say was not coherent.

"What do you mean Sam is being discharged tomorrow?" I asked.

"What are you talking about? What are you really trying to say to me?" I asked again. My brain was freezing up and the motor was sputtering. It seemed that my brain and speech system were not connecting on the path out to connect with the universe. But, it also seemed that my reception was also faulty. I could not understand what I was hearing. Or at least what I thought I was hearing. Was I hallucinating? Was there someone else on the line speaking those words about Sam being discharged from the psychiatric ward tomorrow? Was I really hearing this right?

"Yes, Sam is being discharged tomorrow and you need to come pick him up," Roderick said.

unpredictability
unstable services

"Huh?" I asked. I pushed my ear further into the phone's ear-piece to better hear what Roderick had just said. My brain, thoughts, and speech were topsy-turvy. Was my hearing going haywire as well?

"What? What are you talking about? Who is this?" I insisted.

"Gary. Doc. Dr. Gary. You know this is Roderick. This is Roderick. Did you forget? I am the clinician now working with Sam. Did you forget who I am?" he asked.

"This is Roderick. I am the clinician working with Sam and he is ready for discharge. Certainly, you remember me. I have met you before. Last year when Sam was here I took care of him when he was on the ward. Don't you remember me? I worked with you last year in the emergency room. Of course, I am assigned to the psychiatric unit in the emergency room. Remember?"

"Don't you remember? I worked mostly weekends on the second shift. I am tall and thin. I have rimless glasses that you liked and asked me where I got them. But then you said you needed bifocals and that the lens would be too small to have the bifocals in them. Don't you remember?"

"I told you to go bicycling with the other doctors when you were talking about needing to get more physical activity into your day. You said you needed to exercise more. But then you were also saying that you get enough exercise because you were running around working in the emergency room all day. But then again that physical activity is unfocused. I have worked with you before. I have also worked with Sam before. If you saw me you probably would remember. I am Roderick, the licensed clinical social worker. I am Roderick. Don't you remember?"

He was talking a mile a minute. His speech was not pressured but the words were coming out of his mouth very quickly. My own brain needed antifreeze, reanimation, jump-starting. The memory of him was just not clicking. My brain was short circuiting and it was rebelling. I still could not place him even after all the triggers he gave me.

Anyway, had he paused to take a breath? He was talking in rapid succession. He had just kept on talking. I didn't hear him pause once in his soliloquy to see if I had something to say or ask. Did he even care that I should be part of the conversation? He blithered on, and did not bother to think that I was on the other end of the call.

"Huh? You are Roderick? Yeah. Sure. Okay. What happened to Mei-Lee?" I asked.

"Mei-Lee is now working on another psychiatric ward for the next two weeks, so I took over her caseload," Roderick replied.

"Well, how does any of that make sense?" I finally asked. My brain stopped sputtering and revved into activity.

"Well," I started slowly to make certain that now that my brain seemed to be working that it would stay charged and moving.

"Well, Sam is not ready for discharge," I said emphatically.

"I just saw Sam last night and he was talking gibberish and saying that he is "not going to make it this year." He was way back in the past. He was talking about events that happened twenty or thirty years ago, and none of what he was saying made any sense. If I had been present at those events, the way he was recalling it was not the way I remembered it. Some of the events that he was talking about never happened. I was there, I should know. He was out of his mind. His thought patterns were not coherent. What he was saying made no sense to me. I am sure that if you had spoken to Sam yesterday that it would not make any sense to you either." I said.

"So how can he be ready for a discharge home?" I asked.

"Well the utilization nurse came by yesterday and said that we have to discharge him," Roderick said.

"How's that?" I asked.

"Well, he is not suicidal. He is not saying that he will harm himself. He is not a risk to anyone. He has not harmed anyone before this," Roderick added.

"So, how about the stories and the things that he was telling me yesterday and all last week? What about all that other stuff that he was saying?" I asked.

"I was there last night. My mother was there too," I said.

"He had that wild look in his eyes. His eyes were focused on something outside himself. It would be as if you waved your hands in front of his face that he would not respond. It was if he was not there, present physically, but blank. Just completely blank. You could see that he was distracted. He seemed to be responding to something that only he could hear or see," I said.

"I can confidently tell you that when he looks like that, that he was hearing voices. I can tell you when he is like that, he is not back to reality and back to baseline. I know that he was having auditory hallucinations and hearing voices," I said.

"Well, we need to discharge him," Roderick said.

"His insurance will not pay for him to stay here in the psychiatric unit any longer," Roderick said.

"Well, what's your name? Er, uh, Rod, Roderick, you are the clinician, what do you think?" I asked.

"What did Dr. Ramtell have to say about this?" I asked.

"I know he does not agree with you," I added.

"Well, no. Dr. Ramtell says that Sam might need more time here and that his medications need more adjustment. If we can do that, then we can get Sam near to his baseline. So, so, while it is not ideal, it's probably okay for Sam to go home," Roderick said.

Wired for Sanity

I remembered when I was the doctor helping with the anesthesia for a patient who was going to get electroconvulsive therapy, ECT. I placed the mask over the patient's face and gave the necessary medications. In no time the patient was unconscious. I placed the tube in the throat so that the patient would be under general anesthesia.

We were giving the ECT, or shock treatments as it is commonly known, because he was depressed and had been in the hospital for a long time. He was tried on several medications, nothing seemed to be working, and this was meant to be a boost to get him better faster. The shock treatments were not as in the past when we did not give general anesthesia, and patients experienced memory loss, or had broken bones from the force of the muscle contractions.

While on the psychiatric ward, Sam had the treatments done, and it seemed to get him back closer to the positive side of sanity. But he still had a long way to go, and he was nowhere near baseline then. He seemed really depressed and nothing seemed to work. He had gone through that twice before. While the ECT helped in his recovery, it was not like a light switch, off one minute and then on the next. It took time to see the effects and it would not happen overnight.

Now this time, I saw Sam every day and he was near baseline, but not at baseline. So when Roderick started to tell me about discharge I was confused.

Roderick was speaking in that quiet, calming, reassuring, and non-threatening tone that clinicians tend to use. They and other professionals use that tone when they are trying to reassure you. They are trained to de-escalate conflicts and regain control in a conversation. That manner and tone was an excellent tool to use in any communication, and an essential behavior to prevent and simmer confrontations.

I recognized the habit well as I was also trained to do the same. It was very useful to do to calm angry patients and customers. In any service industry or general conversation it was good to remain calm and reassuring. The manner and tone was supposed to work.

But, right now it was having the opposite effect on me. First, my brain was freezing. Then it was stammering and not working. Finally, it had been fibrillated by a shock that was not meant for me. Now, I felt that I had been electrocuted. The soothing and re-engagement tactic only revved my physical being more. It had accidentally gotten my blood boiling.

To add insult to injury, I was really exhausted. I had been through a terrible shift in the emergency room the night before. When I looked forward, I realized that I was due to go back to work another twelve-hour shift in less than three hours. This meant that I would not get any sleep whatsoever in the next fifteen hours.

I interrupted Roderick just as he began to tell me something else.

"Near baseline and at baseline are two different animals. You are telling me that he is being discharged?" I asked again.

Now I had the opportunity to practice a calming, reassuring manner and tone. This manner was meant to de-escalate conflict and create a win-win for everyone, right? Well, let's test it.

"Well, Rod, let me tell you this," I said very dryly.

"Sam is not anywhere near his baseline. He is hearing voices and seeing things. I know him better than you do. Sam's thoughts are all over the place. If Sam's medications still need adjustment, you have to keep him there to do it. Or, you have to transfer him to someplace, a lower level of clinical care where that can be done. That place, my friend, is not home," I said.

"In any case, even if I agreed with you that he can be discharged, it can't happen today. I have to work for twelve hours in the emergency room less than three hours from now. Since I don't even agree with the discharge home, we should start to think about a plan B," I said.

"Let's think about what you are proposing for him to come home today," I said.

"I won't be home and cannot give him his medications tonight. You know very well that I am the sole caretaker. My mother is at home too. She is an old woman. She cannot do this and she should not have to do it. Anyway, in this state he won't take the medications from her. He will become suspicious and paranoid. He will think that something is up and that she is giving him the wrong medications, if he even takes them at all. They will just end up arguing. That will only make the situation more stressful for him and everyone else. When he is in this bad of a shape, he will only take them from me or from a nurse or the doctor. We can stand there patiently and not budge until he takes them. I don't think she can handle that. It's nerve wracking to stand there and simply wait for Sam to take the pills, and then you have to be certain that he has swallowed them. There is that fine line between being concerned, overbearing, and nagging him to take the pills. My mother can't do that. She is not a health care professional trained to deal with all of that," I said.

"So, tell you what," I said.

My voice was now more calm, clipped, staccato, and very proper. I wanted to communicate clearly to be understood. I wanted Roderick to appreciate and to take into consideration my point of view. That way, he could mull over in his own mind what he intended to do and to think about the consequences of his actions on all the parties involved. Was the proposal in the best interest of the patient? How about the family? Should we even consider the interests of the hospital? Is there even a larger question for his community and society?

I cleared my throat so that the frog that had settled there would jump away.

"Roderick," I began. My voice steadied and I felt I was making the right decision and communicating that effectively to Roderick.

"There must be a better option than the one you gave me. Sam has been living with me for over ten years now, so I think I have a good sense of when he is well, and when he is not. Discharging Sam today is the wrong decision," I said.

I started to think about the case last night that had my nerves on edge and left me so irritated all day. The lack of sleep had not helped and I was tired and left with no reserve after the shift last night. I was running on near empty.

When Roderick called to tell me that Sam was ready for discharge home, I could not take on more stress as I was physically tired and any more demands on me would be too much to bear for that day. I had been trying to suppress the migraine that was swelling in my head.

I intended to create the action plan for a better discharge if Roderick had not done one. It could not be a discharge to home right now and there were other alternatives, right?

Stepping Stone

When Sam was discharged from the psychiatric ward, I could not take him back home at that point. He still needed twenty-four hours of supervised care. Roderick had arranged for him to go to a residential program. It was good that Sam could go there. Sam still needed help after a month stay on the psychiatric ward where he was because of a low point in his illness and his feeling suicidal. I was working twelve hour shifts in the emergency room and could not provide the constant care that he needed at that point. At least, there was staff to help with social activities, and a case manager to work closely with the clinicians in the partial hospital programs, with the hospital, and with the community therapists. The program had its own van and could take Sam out for social and recreational activities, shopping, and errands. My schedule did not allow me to do that so that he could have some semblance of a normal life.

I went to visit Sam on the campus and needed time to re-energize after a particularly contentious meeting with him. He was irritable, negative, and talking about wanting to end his life. I left there that day and I wanted to understand why after so many centuries of information about mental illness there was still a stigma and no cure anywhere in sight.

One of the first hospitals to exclusively treat mental illness opened in the early 1800's. Yet almost two hundred years later, we still do not have an answer or a cure for mental illness. Could this be possible? With other medical problems, like diabetes and asthma, we have come a long way to understand what causes it, and how to treat it. How could we live our best life possible, if our mental health life was out of balance? It was great that many people got to successful recovery, but we had to find a better way, and to clear a path to a cure.

I was feeling more optimistic as I walked out into the warm sun and letting it beat down to recharge my battery. I went to visit Sam every day and he was making steady progress. Then, almost two weeks later, Roderick and Marcie called to tell me that Sam was ready to be discharged home. Marcie was one of the staff persons at the residential program who provided structure, prepared the meals, and helped with social activities.

Each of the clients had their own rooms and Sam had a room on the second floor. When I went to get his things for discharge, the room was a mess. Though his mind was clearer, he was hoarding old magazines, newspaper clippings, empty candy wrappers, and other odd items that he just picked up off the street or around the campus. I hated to burn bridges and did not want to leave the room in that state. Caring for Sam and me was a journey. I knew that at some point I would have to come back here and ask for more help. I tried to get in the habit of not ticking people off.

I was still feeling hopeful. If I were to come back and ask for help, I did not want the staff to have a bad impression of who Sam or I were. I was off the next day from the emergency room. So, refueled by optimism, I found the janitor's closet, took a garbage bag, a bucket and mop, and cleaned the room. I wanted to leave the place neat and clean. Besides, tossing that junk into the garbage bag and cleaning the room was therapeutic, like ridding my attic of things I had not used for five years or longer. It was like a congestion that had to be relieved. I felt like relieving that congestion in the attic relieved the congestion in my own mind. Cleaning the room was therapeutic and I hoped and prayed for sanity to fill the place of the void that was created by tossing out all that junk.

CHAPTER 19

THE OPEN MOUTH

The following day at work, I walked out the trauma room after the surgeons had taken care of an elderly woman who had fallen down a flight of basement stairs. She struck her head and was found semi-conscious at home.

Her neighbors tried to reach her all day. When they could not reach her, they called the police who came and broke the door down. When they went inside she was not in the living room or dining room on the first floor. The door to the basement was open, and they looked there, and saw her at the bottom of the landing. Her head was on the last step, and the rest of her body was a tangled mess, crumpled on the cold basement floor. Her eyes were closed. They spoke to her, she opened her eyes, and she opened her mouth just long enough to say that her hips were hurting. She was bleeding from a cut to her head, and somewhere else on her arms and legs. She had been there all night lying in her own urine and feces.

The emergency medicine technicians moved in and secured her neck with a plastic neck collar. They put bandages to the head wound and took her

235

treat
med injuries
w/ dignity

understaffed?

blood pressure. The paramedics retrieved the longboard from the ambulance and gingerly got her into a position to log-roll her onto the board. In this way they could transport her on the stretcher to the hospital. They did what they could to remove the soiled garments.

It was better to get her up the staircase on the longboard, and then to put her on the stretcher. Once on the landing back on the first floor, they placed the bundle on the stretcher. Though you could adjust the height of the stretcher to accommodate getting persons on or off, or even for the examiner, it would not have been wise to try to get the stretcher up the stairs with her on it. The house did not have a walk out basement, but only a hatch-door. It would be a complete waste of time to find the keys to the hatch-door, to bring the stretcher to the back of the house, and to exit that way. The longboard was solid plastic and could support her weight to get her up the stairs and around corners.

While in the trauma room her skin was oozing from everywhere as her skin was paper thin. She was on a blood thinner and she was bleeding from everywhere. We stabilized her, reversed the blood thinner, and sent her off to have CAT scans from head to toe.

I was not out the trauma room for even a minute, and I did not have time to complete any of my charting in there. As a result, if she did not come back to the emergency room from the CAT scan suite, the clerk would be calling me on my phone and getting on my case that the surgical floor immediately needed my notes. I was figuring out how I was going to catch up with all that when the patient in Room 23 started to scream at the top of her lungs. There was a break in the noise, and less than a minute later she was screaming again.

I walked by Room 23 and stopped to talk to Hanako, who was seated at the nursing station by the rooms at this section of the emergency room. Hanako was hastily tapping into the computer's keyboard and reading the monitor's screen. She tapped again, scrolling rapidly from screen to screen. She appeared to be searching for some specific information.

"What is the matter with Room 23?" I asked.

Hanako looked up from the monitor's screen. She got up from her chair, put kept tapping and scrolling. She apparently had not found the information that she needed just yet. She rested one bent knee on the chair, and put her hand on the back of the chair to prevent it from rolling. She looked as if she was ready to sprint in any minute if needed, or to go back to looking up the information that she was searching.

"Oh, she came in complaining of belly pains and diarrhea," Hanako said.

"Really, and she has to be screaming like that?" I asked.

"That's what I said," Hanako said. "When was the last time that diarrhea caused you to scream like that? Unless of course, you saw an alien coming out in your diarrhea. Then I would really be screaming," Hanako said, and chuckled thinking about the sight of what she just imagined.

"The last time that I heard any screaming like that from a woman it was because she was in labor," Hanako said.

"I know, I know. It surely sounds that way," I said. "Alien diarrhea? I would not want to have that problem either."

"So, is she pregnant?" I asked.

"No," Hanako said.

"How long has she been here in the emergency room?" I asked.

"Oh, only like five minutes. The charge nurse brought her straight back to Room 23. She was screaming too much in the waiting room, and she was scaring the other patients. I was getting scared too. The other patients out there thought that she was out of her mind. They only thought so. I think she has to be out of her mind to be screaming like that just from a little diarrhea. Doesn't she have kids? She should be used to diarrhea by now," Hanako said.

"Well, did she pee? Did we get her urine to see if she is pregnant?" I asked.

"She told the charge nurse and me that her LMP—last menstrual period—was on Sunday. She says she is not pregnant. She insisted that she can't be pregnant," Hanako said.

"Really, and you believe that?" I asked.

"Well, you know me. I told her that if she does not pee, and give me that urine sample in less than five minutes, I will "cath" her for the specimen," Hanako said.

"She will love that. She will love you placing that 16-French catheter into her bladder to get the urine specimen. In fact, show her the 28-French catheter that is much bigger. That should scare her enough for her to pee in less than two minutes flat. That tactic usually works. Guaranteed," I said with sarcasm.

"Yeah, yeah. I really was not going to do that, but scare tactics sometimes work. But, I have a plan B, just in case. I drew blood to see if she is pregnant, but that will not come back right away," Hanako said.

A bloodcurdling scream exploded from the room, and it was longer this time. The little hair that I had left on my scalp rose straight up. That screaming was straight out of the *Exorcist*, and my body quivered from the sound.

"Let's go see what's up with her," I said.

Hanako and I walked into the room, and I looked at the patient.

"Hi, Miss, I am Dr. Gary and this is Hanako, but you met her already," I said.

I pulled my badge forward so that she could clearly see my name and the title that I was the doctor. The name badge was tethered on the trinket badge-holder with the hospital's logo on it. I had to make sure that I did that so that the patient knew who I was. I always clearly identified myself so that the patients knew who was taking care of them. Besides, I wanted to have good customer service scores. The last thing I wanted was for some patient to say that they had no clue who the doctor was who took care of them, or that they never even saw a doctor. And that *Dr. Marcus Welby* stuff where "you look like a doctor, so you must be a doctor" does not fly here.

"Yes, I am Dr. Gary," I repeated.

The name badge now snapped back in place against the upper left pocket of my white lab-coat.

"We are here to take care of you," I said.

"What seems to be the matter?" I asked.

"I am having diarrhea," the patient said.

"Oh? When did it start?" I asked.

"Oh, just now. Just now, today, a minute ago," the patient said.

"Oh? But it seems like something else is wrong, and that you are having strong belly pains," I said.

"What else is going on?" I asked.

"Are you pregnant? When was your last menstrual period?" I asked, trying to hide the hint of disbelief in my voice that she was not pregnant.

"I had my menstrual period on Sunday," the patient said.

"Sunday, as in six days ago?" I now asked, the pitch of my voice rising and erasing the trace of disbelief. With the way I had ended the sentence with a higher pitch she must have known that this was a question, even if the hint had now given way to my strong disbelief.

"Yes. Yes, it was on Sunday," the patient said.

"Are you certain, Sunday?" I asked, making sure that I was speaking slowly and clearly and the pitch rising so that she knew this was really a question I was asking. Was she really not pregnant and I was imagining that her rounded belly was something else? An ovarian tumor or some other type of problem in her belly? Excess weight in the midsection did not generally look like that. Had I become that clueless?

"Yes, it was last Sunday, one week ago. I know my own body," said the patient.

I looked at Hanako standing on the other side of the bed. Hanako stared at me and rolled her eyes. She did not believe the patient either.

"And the one before that?" I asked, now more calmly than with the questions before.

"One month ago," she confidently replied.

"Huh? And it was normal?" I asked with my left eyebrow crinkling and going upward as I started to frown.

"Uhm." My lips were tight, puckered, and twisted in the opposite direction of the left eyebrow, and to the right.

Hanako rolled her eyes again. This time I was certain that I saw into Hanako's cranium as she rolled her eyes so high in their sockets in obvious disbelief of what the patient was saying.

"Uhm," I again said to no one in particular.

I looked over at the patient again, and looked at her abdomen.

"Uhm?"

If that was not a gravid, pregnant, abdomen, well I will be darned.

"Are you sure? You look like you are pregnant," I said.

"Have you been pregnant before?" I asked. If she had been pregnant before she must have known what that experience was like. I assumed that that was not an experience that the memory would completely suppress and could not readily recall.

"Yes. I have a son who is two years old," the patient said.

"Are you sexually active?" I quizzed her some more. What she was telling me made absolutely no sense what-so-ever to me.

"Yes, I am married," said the patient.

"Is your husband here with you today?" I asked.

"No, he is in Patterson," said the patient.

"Patterson? As in the state of New Jersey?" I asked.

"Yes," said the patient.

"Oh. Okay. Do you mind if I take a look at your belly?" I asked.

"Sure, no problem," the patient said.

I moved closer to the bed to take a look at her belly and to examine it. I intended to continue to ask more questions, but not wanting to waste too much more time. Hanako pulled one side of the sheet down and I pulled the other side.

That's meconium. That was meconium and it smelled like it. That was not diarrhea. Meconium is the baby's bowel movement and it sure smelled like stool. Just before Hanako or I could say anything else, the patient made the last scream and immediately from between her legs the head of the baby popped into the bed.

"Oh, Oh!" Hanako and I yelled together.

"Well. Well. You are pregnant," I said. Our reflexes were quick and our movements purposeful with every muscle memory kicking into high gear. The baby was small enough that it came out with that last contraction. I quickly turned the baby over, and yelled for Hanako to get the baby suction bulb out of the drawer. I had to clear out the mouth, the throat, and the nose at once before it inhaled any of that poop. Hanako pulled opened the top drawer to get the pediatric nasal bulb, and I immediately cleared the baby's mouth, throat, and nose of any of it.

"Help! Help in 23!" I yelled out to anyone in the hallway, and Hanako slammed the call-light button. When the secretary answered to ask how she could help, Hanako screamed that we needed the pediatrician and obstetricians, OBs, in 23, STAT.

"STAT! We had a precipitous delivery in Room 23. Call it over ahead and tell them to come SUPER STAT!" I said.

But, that was only the start. I would have to put a tube into the throat to clear any meconium out. One of the nurses outside must have heard the desperate shout for help and rushed into the room with the pediatric crash cart. We also needed to keep the baby warm by wrapping her up. In no time, the pediatricians and OBs would be here, and I knew that the neonatologist would come with an incubator to keep the baby warm.

"Look at that! She was pregnant!" I said.

"No kidding!" Hanako said with her eyes still rolling.

As quickly as the commotion started, it died down. I was used to that rapid spike in adrenaline one minute, then down to the baseline all within five minutes or less. It was like that at home with Sam too, so I learned that this too shall pass, and I took in gulps of air, and breathed deeply.

The baby was whisked away by the neonatologists and we were left with the patient trying to understand what had just happened as our job was done for the baby. The patient looked up at me and Hanako and apologized saying, "Thank you for saving my baby."

But my pulse and my heart beating fast against my chest were not yet back to normal. I still felt every beat as it thumped right up to my rib cage and kicked the ribs on the upstroke. I sighed and smiled. Yes, she was pregnant. A migraine was starting to form, and I remembered Simone when we were kids—"Make it come through my mouth."

"Doc, please take it from my mouth," Simone screamed. In the midst of my migraine I heard the phrase over and over again. Pregnancy was not an easy condition to bear. Simone was pregnant when we were mere kids, and she was only thirteen years old then. Didi came home laughing, not because Simone was pregnant, but because Simone was asking them to take the baby from her mouth. Didi was grown at eighteen years old and knew everything. She laughed saying that Simone was asking for the baby to come through her mouth. Didn't everyone know where babies came from? But the contractions were so bad that Simone just wanted a way out of her pain. It was not that she did not know where babies came from. When you are in a crisis, who knows what you will say or do.

"Make it come through my mouth. Please, doctor, take it from my mouth, doctor."

Didi said that Simone's mother was "as mad as a hatter" because she did not know that Simone was pregnant. No one knew, and apparently not even Simone. But she must have. In retrospect, that's why Simone started to wear loose clothing and sweat-pants, and we only thought she was gaining weight. So when the labor pains started she had no idea what was going on.

At that time in the emergency room, the doctors told Simone's mother that Simone was pregnant, and about to deliver the baby. Simone's mother turned beet red from embarrassment and from shame. How could she not know that Simone was pregnant? She saw her every day and she lived in the same house. How could she not have known? Did she not feel the intuition?

However, right now, Simone's mother could not think clearly to understand her own ignorance of the event that now lay before her. But in any case, she was determined to hold her head up and not die from fear and shame. She remembered her grandmother always saying to her, "Shame will kill you! Pride goeth before destruction! Don't be stopped by shame. Always do the right thing, and take responsibility for your actions. Stand up and do the right thing, but don't die from shame!"

Nonetheless, at that point Simone's mother simply said, "Deliver the baby, doctor, and we will cope with it."

"Make it come through my mouth," Simone screamed again.

"We will deliver the baby now, but why don't you wait in the family room," the doctor said.

"By the way, she will probably need to talk to a psychiatrist and a therapist," the doctor added.

"Yes, Doctor, that is a good idea. Do you think I should talk to them too?" Simone's mother asked, as she was not really sure what to do, and where to start next.

"Yes. That's a very good idea," the doctor said. "It would help for both of you to talk to someone. You will have a lot to talk about, I am sure."

In the midst of that memory, I realized that sometimes to get through an unbearable pain you prayed that there was another way to get to a happy end, but in a path that was not as intensely painful. Some people use drugs, alcohol, or sex to medicate the pain. But when you are most vulnerable, you probably won't make the best choices, and the consequences may be disastrous.

I glanced at Hanako, and we both smiled at the patient thankful that the baby seemed to be all right for now. The woman started to express her thanks to us. She blushed and started to cry.

"Oh, you are welcome, my friend," I said.

"Yes. You are welcome," Hanako added.

Dr. Emily Rivers, the OB-GYN resident, went out the door behind the transporters who came to take the patient to Labor and Delivery to get her admitted. The senior doctor, Dr. Tiffany Williams, the specialist in high-risk pregnancies, lingered a minute or two in the doorway. She dealt with the pregnancies where the mother had other problems like high blood pressure, heart and lung problems, diabetes, drug use, and mental health problems.

"No matter what you do, do not let her leave this hospital until she is seen by psychiatry," I said, while pulling on Dr. Williams' jacket sleeve.

"No doubt, no doubt," Dr. Williams said.

"We see this too often nowadays, and you will be surprised about what we learn is going in the woman's life why she denies what is an obvious pregnancy," she added. "Besides, there is also the problem of post-partum depression, with women being sad and in the "dumps" after the baby is born."

"I have no intention whatsoever to have this mother leave the hospital without being seen by psychiatry. At least not on my watch," Dr. Williams said.

"Thank you, thank you," Hanako and I both said together.

Williams turned and walked down the hallway to catch up with the patient and her resident. Hanako and I both breathed sighs of relief. Yes, my nerves had been raw all day, and my heart was still beating a little bit too fast.

I was a bit irritated too. How could she not know she was pregnant? She had been pregnant before. What did she think it was that must have been moving and kicking in her abdomen? How could she not know she was pregnant? Was it because she did not want to be in that state? Where was the husband? What was his story anyway?

Small White Pill

"What medications are you taking Mr. Solomon?"

"Oh, I don't know. I take a small white pill, a large white one, and a medium orange one," he said.

"How many pills do you take, sir, only three, or more than three?" I asked.

"I take five tablets every day," he said.

"So, what are the names of the pills?" I asked.

"I don't know. You should know," Mr. Solomon said.

"Well, how is that?" I asked now completely confused. Had I in fact seen him before and should know what medications he was taking?

"Well, you are the doctor, you should know what I am taking," he confidently responded.

"Mr. Solomon, I am the emergency room doctor. I am Dr. Gary," I said to remind him who I was.

"You told me your doctor is Dr. Connor on Weymouth Drive. I don't think I have ever seen you as a patient, have I?" I asked him getting myself even more confused. I was wracking my brain to remember if I had seen him before.

"Well," I thought to myself, "if he has been to this hospital before, there is information in the electronic medical record that I could look up to confirm his medications and past medical history."

I glanced again at the summary sheet the nurse gave me. The demographic sheet would reveal if he had been here before. It would have his medications, allergies, medical history, and who he told us was his primary care doctor. I looked at it before I came into the room, and was sure that he had not been here before. The nurse had question marks by medications. He did not know the names, and apparently she could not figure it out either.

"You are the doctor. You should know what the small and large white pills are, and what the orange one is," he said again.

"It's in your computer system. The nurses and doctors always put that information in their system when I go to them," he said.

"I understand that. But, let me try to explain why we don't have it," I said.

"You go to another hospital. That information is in their computer system. We are not the same hospital."

"You are now at this hospital's emergency room. We do not have any information about you in our computer system. We have no record of you being here, and I don't have access to your records," I said.

"Well, you are the doctor, you should know," he said.

"Anyway, that makes no sense to me," he added.

"Uh…," I muttered. I agreed with what was the obvious.

"That hospital across town is less than two miles from this hospital, right?" he asked. He was making more a statement of fact, rather than asking me a question, therefore, I nodded in agreement.

"Dr. Connor has this information in her computer system, and it's in their computer too."

"You have a computer system but yet it's not in yours," he said.

"Why don't the two computers talk to each other?" he asked. His eyebrows were turned up to make a question mark.

His eyebrows implied the question, "Yeah, stupid, why don't the computers connect and talk to each other?"

I sighed, and said, "Sadly, they do not. This hospital is on one system, and that hospital is on another. We are not one hospital system, and the information does not cross over," I said.

"Well, that's dumb," he said.

I smiled and nodded in agreement.

I liked him already as he was a straight talker. There was no mumbo jumbo, and he got to the point very quickly.

"My son is working in China and I Skype him there all the time," he said.

"I can talk to him right now if I want from this cell phone he gave me with one phone call."

"I can even see him and talk to him at the same time, just like I am talking to you now, face to face."

"I thought you doctors were smart," he said. I laughed. He was a real comedian.

"Well, in some things we are smart, and in other things, not so much," I said.

"But we are working on it," I said.

"But look. It's now eleven o'clock at night. Dr. Connor's office is now closed."

"Let me call the pharmacy chain and they can tell me what medications you are on," I said and laughed again.

"What pharmacy do you use?" I asked.

"Hopefully, it is one that you go to all the time and I could get a complete record of the medications," I said.

"Oh, it's the one on Mabel Street. It's open all night," he said.

"Great. I will go call them and be back in a minute," I said.

"We are in luck; the pharmacy had a complete listing of your medications, including all your allergies."

I wrote them out for him on a piece of paper that was small enough for him to keep in his wallet for future reference.

I smiled and said, "May I make a suggestion, Mr. Solomon?"

"Go ahead."

"The computers should talk to each other, but right now they don't. But we are working on it. Your pharmacy and your doctor have your medical records."

"Right."

"It's good for you to have a backup plan. First, you should know all the names of the medications that you are taking and what you are taking them for."

He nodded.

"Remembering them all in your head is hard," I said.

Remembering all the meds was hard and I knew what that was like. Sam was on several medications too. I kept a list with me so that I can tell the ambulance and the health care workers what the doses are. Sam had been on Lithium, Depakote, and Lasix. Some medications needed blood levels drawn regularly, and careful watching of several things, for example, the red and white cell counts, and the liver and kidney functions. Frequently, the doses of the meds had to be adjusted. Some doses went up and down depending on the situation. Keeping the information up to date and writing them down was very helpful. It was one fewer thing to worry about in an emergency when you are too tired, too stressed or not able to think quite right because too much was going on all at once around you.

"Mr. Solomon, while we are working on getting all the computers connected so that they speak to each other, this is what you can do to help yourself and help us better help you."

"Write the names, the doses, and how often you take the pills on a piece of paper, and keep that in your wallet. You can also put your medical conditions, and any person who you want us to call for you in case of an emergency on the same paper, if you like. You may consider getting a medical alert bracelet to put your medical problems and allergies on it too."

"Do you have any questions so far?" I asked to make sure he was following me, and I could explain more if he wanted me to. He said that he had none.

"Each time you go to the doctor or pharmacy or hospital ask them to update the sheet for you or give you a card with all that information on it," I said.

"You could also put all your medicine bottles, including any vitamins, herbal supplements, or any over-the-counter medications you are taking in a bag. Bring them with you each time you go to the doctor so that they can go over them with you."

"Do you have any questions so far?" I asked.

"No. I will keep this sheet and ask Dr. Connor to go over it with me," he said chuckling.

"Are you sure that is okay and you don't have questions?" I asked.

"Well, uh, you know, Dr. Connor does go over all my medicines with me each time I see her. Uh, but most times I don't even listen. I see her put information in the computer too. So I figured you and all your computers know what I take."

"That's all right," I said.

"Do this as a backup, and keep the list with you so that the next time you can tell us the pills you take."

"Does that sound good?" I asked.

"Good," he said.

"Now, what was troubling you to bring you to the emergency room tonight?" I asked.

"My blood sugar reading has been running very high and I am worried about it," he said.

"You see, I am a diabetic," he said.

"Oh," I said and stopped to ask him some questions about that.

An Unusual Problem

Mariek leaned on the door frame while holding a chart in her hand.

"So, which one of you is the lucky one to see the patient in Room 20?" she asked with a smirk on her face. She was twirling her pen and flicking it back and forth thinking, "I have all the time in the world, so none of you can dodge this one this time."

"So, which one of you is the lucky one today?" she asked again as sweetly as possible.

We pretended as if we had not heard her, and kept on looking at the computer screens in front of us since she was lounging on the door and twirling her pen as if she were handling a toy and playing a game.

She was asking so sweetly to cajole a volunteer from among the doctors. Whoever and whatever was in that room must be unique, quite different from the norm, but it could not have been a true emergency. Otherwise, Mariek would just have grabbed onto any lab-coat sleeve and pulled us off the chairs.

You can catch flies with honey, and since none of us took the bait, eventually, Mariek just said, "Well, Dr. Rubenstein just did the last one. Dr. Omoleke did the one before, and Dr. Roshni did them all yesterday. So, Dr. Gary, this one goes to you."

The other doctors tightened their bodies, rounded up their shoulders, and moved in closer to the computers as if they had to go inside the machines to see, to read, and to understand what was on the screens in front of them.

All of that did not make them look any smaller or inconspicuous either. It was classic avoidance behavior, and Mariek simply ignored all that with us trying to look small, busy, and not hearing too well. It was like being in a high school class and the students silently praying, "Teacher, don't call on me, please God, don't let her call on me, I don't know the answer, and I don't want to look like a fool in front of everyone."

Mariek simply ignored all that posturing, walked into the room, and dropped the chart and information on my hand as I was clicking on the mouse to the computer.

"Dr. Gary, Room 20 is yours. It's your turn."

I looked up at her quizzically. When did people become so bold, and just dropped work in your lap that you obviously did not want to do, and did not volunteer for? Could Mariek not have interpreted all the avoidance cues I was showing, and know that I was not interested, and no amount of work ethic could be marshaled to get me to go see the patient in Room 20? Her behavior told me it was not an emergency, and it probably was not all that urgent either.

I interpreted her actions as that this would be interesting, very different, and leaving an impression. But, what about my own choice, what if I were not interested? Okay, okay, it was obviously now for me to deal with; therefore, I stood up and walked towards Room 20.

Mariek was at my heels, saying, "Yah, you need a female chaperone for this one, and I am here to help you."

She loved working in the emergency room because it brought in the unexpected, and people from all walks of life. She traveled the world with her military family while growing up, and she thrived on the unusual. Nothing fazed her as she had seen it all and lived it all. She loved people and chatted with them about their families, children, dogs, cats, food, books they had read, movies they had seen—you name it. She loved puzzles and mysteries. But, when she pulled me off my chair to come to the room, she refused to clue me in to what all the cloak-and-dagger behavior was all about. She had not allowed me to look at the computer screen to see the complaint, or to read through the nursing notes that had already been recorded there.

I entered the room, Mariek closed the door behind me, and I looked over to see the patient that was in the room. Mariek had already pulled the pelvic cart into the room, and had taken the necessary supplies out. I guessed the patient's age, and started to think about Mariek's weird behavior. The patient was well dressed, wore a multi-strand white pearl necklace, and had a stunning diamond solitaire on her left ring finger. Why was she in the emergency room so late at night, and why did Mariek refuse to give me any clues?

CHAPTER 20

WHAT'S UP, DOC?

I committed to continue on the path that I was certain was the correct one. The wind said so and I decided to listen to it.

I looked right and I looked left, and when I saw that there were no cars coming right behind me, I made a sharp and narrow U-turn in the road. I stopped behind the ambulance and then jumped out of my car and left the engine still running.

There was a man with one shoe off lying on the grassy knoll outside a bunch of apartments. There was a full moon out, but a passing cloud blocked the natural light for a minute. The sole street light at this part of the grassy field did not provide sufficient lighting to see as clearly as I would have liked. A brisk cold wind was starting to pick up, and I pulled my thin jacket closer around my body. I could not tell if I was being affected by the poor lighting, the gravitational pull of a full moon, or being chilled by the wind. I was filled with fearful anticipation of what I was going to see once I stepped up to the ambulance crew and the man who was just lying there. Was he dead? The man was hardly moving at all.

The man had no coat on and his shirt was jacked up showing part of his belly. He was not paying too much attention to the commotion around him. Was he just lying there happy in whatever substance he had imbibed, or had he already transitioned to the other side?

The ambulance attendant was bent over him, asking "Sir, sir, are you okay? What's your name?" The attendant was trying to bring him back or wake him up. "Wake up," he said, "and tell me what happened. Wake up. I need to check you out. What happened? I am going to take your blood pressure. Tell me, what happened?" the attendant repeatedly said.

Another attendant grabbed her stethoscope and quickly pulled on some latex gloves.

I walked up to them and saw immediately that it was Sam. Who else could it be? Sam looked as if he were sleeping. I stepped up further and interrupted them as they bent over him. Yes, it was Sam.

"I will take care of it."

The male ambulance attendant turned around and looked at me.

"Oh, are you gonna ride with us to the hospital?" The ambulance attendant asked in surprise. He quickly looked at the stranger who had spoken and intervened. Then he grinned when he recognized the stranger that approached him.

"Oh," he said.

"What's up, Doc?" he said.

"Oh, it is you, Dr. Gary. I did not recognize you in civvies, you know, civilian clothes. Where are your tie and lab-coat?"

"Are you not working in the emergency room today?" he asked.

"No. Not today. I am off today. I will be there tomorrow though," I said.

"Yeah, it's me," I said again to be sure that they really recognized me out of my usual work clothes.

"Yeah, I will take care of it," I said emphatically. "No, I am not working the emergency room today," I said. I was unnecessarily repeating myself.

"Do you know this guy?" the attendant asked.

"Yep," I said very tersely. The ice was back.

"It's my brother. I will take care of him and take him home," I said. I was trying to cut the conversation very short, and not trying to do any explanation about why my brother was lying on this grassy field in practically the middle of the night. I was not in the mood to tell him, blow by blow, what was going on, and how we happened to be in this place and at this time and in this circumstance. What would be the use?

"Do you want me to take his blood pressure to make sure it's okay?" the attendant asked.

"No, he is all right," I replied. Sam had to be all right as I had found him and I would figure it out and take care of it. Besides, I had a blood pressure cuff at home. I would be wasting more precious time for the attendant to take the blood pressure. If it was too low, what was I to do anyway? I was not going to go back to the emergency department to have them simply hang a bag of saline to bring the blood pressure back up. That could take all night. If the blood pressure was too high? They would have simply given him the same blood pressure pill he takes at home to bring it down. Then I would be stuck there waiting for them to document in their records what they had done, or not done. They would scribble illegible notes, unless they had an electronic medical record, about the clinical treatment given, and the treatment's effect. Did their treatment work? Was it not six of one, half a dozen of the other? That made no sense for me to waste their time and waste my time to sit there all night. It was unnecessary for them to just monitor him. Could I not do the very same thing at home?

Suddenly, I understood why Sam seemed pleasantly happy, dazed, and not talking too much. I saw the empty bottle of rum by Sam's side. Obviously, the ambulance attendants had not seen it yet.

"Are you sure you don't want me to take his blood pressure?" the attendant asked again just to be sure.

"No, no, I got it," I said to them now with more emphasis. "Please, only help me get him into my car and that will be good," I said.

It took all three of us to get him to his feet. An assist of three. Nurses and techs and aides do this all day—lifting and pulling and assisting and propping and fluffing and cajoling. God bless 'em. And Sam was in no shape to assist. None. Truthfully, a Hoyer lift would have been quite handy now. It would have made it easier to move him rather than trying to lift a body that could not and would not even try to help. It was pure dead weight. Could I get a portable Hoyer lift to put in my trunk for the next time around? But, let there not be a next time. Please.

We got Sam's torso into the car's front seat first, and Sam could not even help with swinging his legs into the car. I grabbed the bottom of his trousers, and used the top half of my body as a fulcrum to leverage and swing the bottom half of his body into the car. I breathed and slammed the car door shut. I would put the seat belt on when I got into the car, and I didn't even bother looking for the other shoe.

"Thanks guys, thanks. You guys are the best. Really. Thanks," I said.

"No problem Dr. Gary, see you soon," they replied.

"Yes, see you in the emergency room soon," I said.

I climbed into the front seat and reached over Sam to put his seat belt on. I then put mine on and turned on the radio. The car's engine was still running, and I reversed from the ambulance and pulled along the side of it, and then took the immediate right on to Nahum Drive to take Sam home.

I glared at Sam. He was so drunk and he had no clue about what was going on.

"You just can't make anything easy, right?" I asked. "Why is everything about you so complicated?"

There was complete silence.

"You promised that you would stop drinking, and I have told you that you cannot mix alcohol with your meds," I said.

"You promised you would stop drinking," I talked into the air. "If you keep this up people will think you are a habitual drunkard," I said.

The therapists claim that people sometimes use alcohol, or drugs, or both, to mask their emotional pain, or to hide other mental illness. But this was too much really. We had gotten him to the point where Sam would take his medications and go to the appointments at the mental health center. This had been the longest period where he had remained relatively stable. At regular periods his mind would unravel, and he would have to be admitted to the psychiatric ward or a psychiatric institution for months. If he had not developed pneumonia and was weakened by that, we would not have been in this place. If he had not needed physical rehab after that bout with pneumonia I would have just taken him back home after that admission. But, he had become debilitated and could not climb the stairs, so I had few options at that point.

Sam must have been in some other place in his own dream. What was I going to do? I tried to reason through a logical course of action. Emotional pain, huh? If you drink and do drugs to mask it, when you wake up the pain and problems are still there, and you will have done nothing to fix the problems. Then what do you have to do, go drinking and drugging some more? I asked the universe. Isn't that just exchanging one demon for another on your back?

"But, finding you now like this on the grass is a better outcome than the usual," I said to myself. If the police had been the ones to find Sam tonight I would have to come get him out of jail or deal with some other nonsense. This was a better outcome that the ambulance found him first.

"Thank you, this was a better outcome than dealing with the police tonight," I repeated.

However, what was I missing? You were doing well, now this. What was I missing? What assumptions had I made that were wrong? It seemed that we had this all wrapped up, right diagnosis, right meds, everything was right? What was wrong, did something change? Were we completely off base? Where do I start again, to figure this all out? Was I wrong to have him at home for the last ten years? Was this a good idea for me, for him, or for anyone else?

The silence in the car was only broken by an occasional snore or gasp from Sam. I drove in silence home hoping that by the time I got home Sam's own two legs would carry him up the stairs. I would have to muster enough strength to get him into the shower and get him cleaned up. This was not the easiest thing that I had ever done. Sam did not make it simple, and he did not make it easy.

"But, whoever promised that they would make anything easy for you?"

No. Life was not easy and it was not meant to be. Life was not easy and I knew with certainty from working in the emergency room that it was not like an afternoon romp in a rose garden.

Not Seeing Eye to Eye

I was in Room 3 in the emergency room when Jennifer and Gordon, two paramedics, came into the room to bring in the elderly patient. They had called ahead to tell us that a code was coming. The patient was not breathing and she had no pulse.

It turned out to be a ninety year-old woman from a nursing home that the nurses had found when they were making their rounds during their shift. After the nurses called the ambulance, and when Jennifer got there, she had asked the nurses to give them a copy of the living will so that they could take it with them to the hospital. In the haste of doing everything, the nurses had not gotten all the paperwork together ahead of time. If they had looked in the chart for information about the advanced directive, it would have revealed what to do if the patient were not breathing or did not have a heart rate. Apparently, the nurses could not find the information. But, the nurses said they would try to reach the family and her doctor to ask them if the woman wanted to be resuscitated and to be on life support.

can't find DNR

Since there was no living will available, Jennifer went ahead and started the resuscitation. She gave the first round of medications and placed the breathing tube into the woman's throat. They continued to pump on the woman's chest and breathed for her through the plastic tube. It only took about seven minutes for them to get to the emergency room and we had already brought the crash cart into the room. We were standing by and ready to continue CPR when they came into the room.

Gordon was pumping on the chest, and Jennifer was squeezing the air bag while pushing the stretcher with her other hand. We transferred the patient off the stretcher with a slide board onto the emergency room bed, and it was one of the new ones where you could do CPR on them.

"Gordon, those are pacemaker spikes on the monitor. She has a pacemaker."

"We knew that's what it was and we saw the bump on the right chest," Jennifer said.

"Hold CPR," I said. I felt for a pulse, and there was none. I felt for a pulse at the neck and listened with my stethoscope over the heart. There was nothing. With no pulse she would not be breathing.

The monitor looked like that there were lots of spikes and artifact. Were we being fooled by the spikes there on the monitor? Was there some kind of heart rhythm and a faint pulse that we could not feel?

"Where is the bedside ultrasound?"

"Let's get it and look quickly at the heart, as I don't think that there is a heartbeat. We have to learn to trust our judgment. That is just extra noise on the monitor, artifact. There is no heartbeat, no pulse, and no blood pressure," I said. "But we will double check to convince ourselves that we are right."

"Where is the bedside ultrasound?" I asked again.

"Oh, I don't know," Ryan said.

"Where is it?" I asked Ryan. He looked at me and shrugged his shoulders. "No one knows?"

"Oh, I am sure it is in Room 2. That's where the last code was," Lisette said. This was the fourth code in less than four hours.

"Well, why did we not put it back in its rightful place?" I asked. Dr. Maurice, the emergency room director ran a tight ship. He was ex-military and he always said to minimize stress in emergencies you have to have a systematic approach to the problem. "Prepare for the unexpected, and the unexpected will be easier to deal with when it comes."

Ryan went to Room 2 to get the ultrasound machine and he came back with it. I placed the plastic sheath over the probe, turned on the machine, and looked at the heart to convince ourselves that the heart was not doing anything. I looked at the monitor with the waves flat-lined interrupted only by spikes from the jolts from the pacemaker. On the ultrasound window the heart was completely still.

"Well, how long have we been doing CPR?" I asked.

"It's been at least fifteen minutes," Jennifer said.

Before I had a chance to say anything more, the door was flung wide open by a man that was upset and protesting whatever the nurse on his heels was trying to say to him. I turned around to face him as the other nurse caught up to him to try to stop him from coming into the room. However, at that point it was too late.

"That's my mother," he said. "That's my mother."

"Who is the doctor in charge?" he asked. I was the only one with a lab-coat on in the room, so tag I am it, no?

"Hi. I am Dr. Gary," I said. "Can you give us a minute, please? I will come out to talk to you in a second."

No sooner had I said that than a woman who was the man's spitting image appeared—she must have been his sister.

"That's my mother," she said. "I want everything done."

"No. She doesn't," the man said. "She does not want you to pump on her chest. She doesn't want to be on life support." The argument escalated between the two about what to do with their mother.

"Well, where is the living will?" I asked. "What does your mother want? It's really your mother's choice."

"Well, I am Mr. Blount. I don't want her resuscitated. I don't want that. She has a living will that says she does not want that."

The brunette beside him shook her head in disagreement.

"That's wrong. I want everything done. I am her daughter and I want everything to be done."

"As I said, it really should be what your mother would want. I am really sorry. We have been doing CPR now for at least fifteen minutes and there has been no response to our efforts. Your mother has passed on. She is gone," I said.

I hated to tell them that in the middle of the room with us at the end of CPR and everyone still in the room. I would have preferred to go to the family room, given them the news, sat with them for a while, answered their questions, and offered them to see pastoral care if they wanted. Who wants to hear that information among all that activity in the resuscitation room?

However, you have to prepare for the unexpected, as well as the expected. Most likely none of them was the legally appointed health care representative, and if one of them was, they would have said so. In a time of crisis and grief, the last thing that you really needed was the family fighting, and you wanted them to be supportive of each other. Once the shock wore off, and you were only left with grief, who wanted to add discontent and a strained relationship into the mix?

Living with Sam, uncertainty was a way of life. To prevent every day from being a bad mental health day, I had to be prepared for the definite life changes. I was Sam's conservator and I had a will. Who would take over and care for Sam if I were not here? I was also fortunate that Sam had not fired me yet as his conservator. I have many friends living with family members with mental illness. They would tell me that they were constantly being fired and re-hired for the job.

Sometimes when that happened it was for the best. It was best to share the load and have someone else take over. Sometimes personalities clash, people change, and for your own mental health it may make sense for another person who can best handle the uncertainty to prepare for it and handle it. The seas ebb and flow, there is high tide and low tide. You did not have to be a hero every day and all day. To help the family member with mental illness first meant that you had to anchor your own self. If you were in a bad frame of mind and there was so much fighting between you, it did make sense to ask a neutral party to step in and help you out for a while. You are better served by asking for help, and the trick was to learn to ask when you really needed it.

TIP BOX 5

1. You are stronger than you believe to make it through life's changes and adversities

2. Plan for the expected life changes: Make a will, a list of your assets, a power of attorney and an advance directive. Think about and plan for who will be the successor to take over your affairs if you are not able to do so

3. Create an emergency medical contact sheet: Include medications, doses, allergies, doctors, and who to call in case of emergency. Keep it in a safe but convenient place. Also keep a copy in your wallet

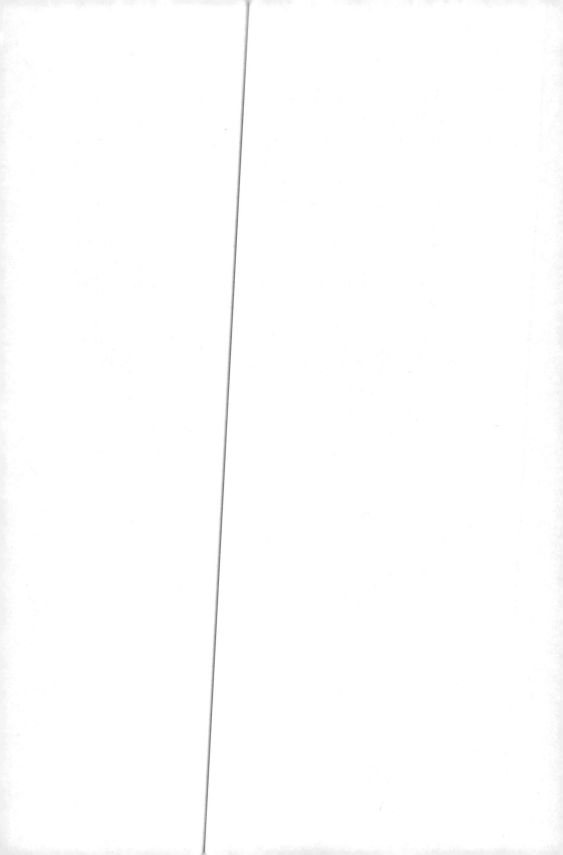

PART VI

SUNNY SKIES

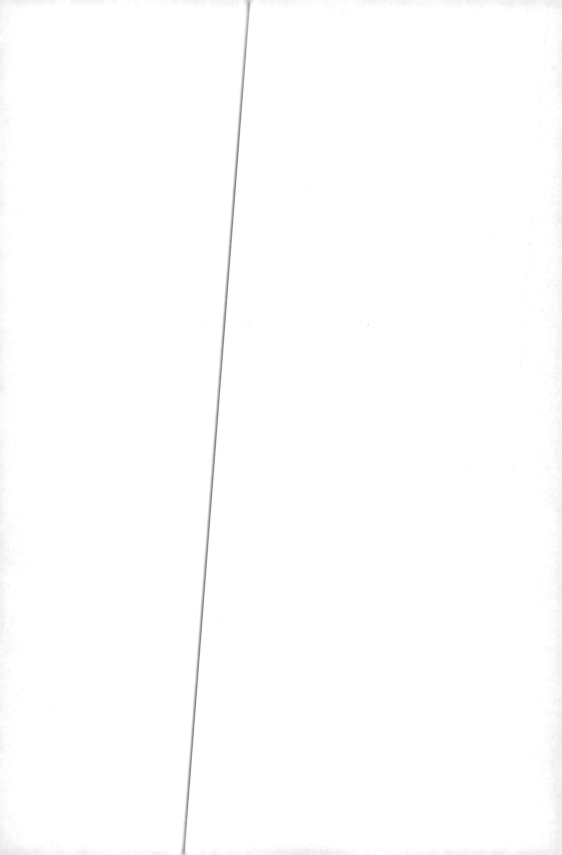

Stepping Stones in the Rose Garden
Silently...
Stepping on stones in the garden's bed
Pruned and plucked
Tweaked and tucked
Dead wood chopped
Shriveled leaves cropped
Lightly...
Thorns bring forth searing pain
Bleeding from the maim
Life flowing freely to create the stain
Of a memory...
Poising on the stepping stone
Reaching here and there
Everywhere...
Unseen hands grooming
A future life you cannot see
Coiffed to near perfection
Contracted to a mere reflection
Of what you used to be...
Crumpled small to preserve
Brought inside out to conserve
To expand the blooms
Roses with untold beauty...

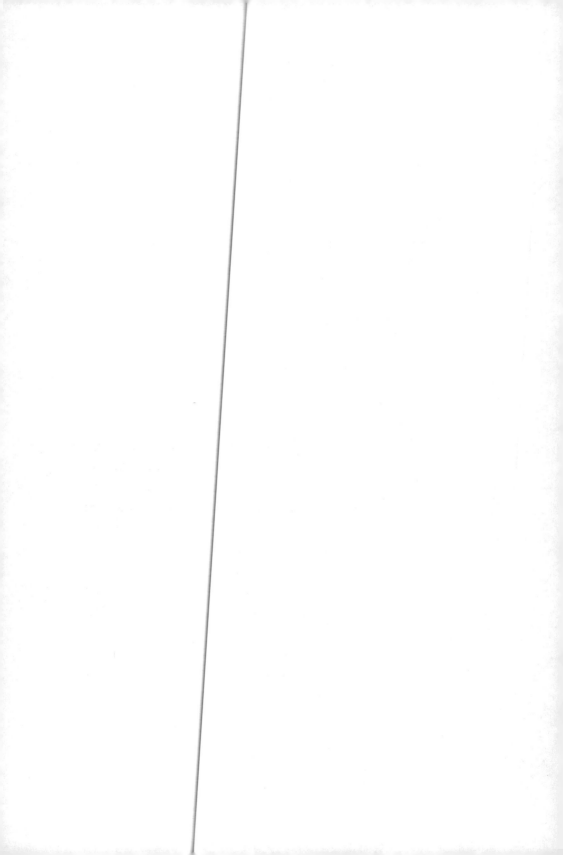

CHAPTER 21

UNANSWERED QUESTIONS

"D r. Hillpoint," I am confused.
"I thought you said that Sam has schizophrenia. The other psychiatrist told me that he has bipolar disorder. That's why he had shock treatments when he was really depressed. It helped for a while but then we were back to square one. Now, you are telling me it's more likely bipolar disorder, rather than schizophrenia?"

"Which is it, schizophrenia, or bipolar disorder, or both?"

"He has had many psychiatrists. When he was first diagnosed years ago, that was what we thought, schizophrenia. Now, I am not so certain. I think after the many years living with the diagnosis of schizophrenia, and as events unfold, it is more likely on a spectrum of bipolar disorder." Hillpoint said.

"How do you treat the problem if you don't know the correct diagnosis? It's like getting to the root cause. You have to know what the problem is to come up with the right treatment."

"Not everything in life is as clear cut as that, Dr. Gary, you know that. When you have lived long enough you know that," Hillpoint said.

"We live in a world of uncertainty. But in this case, I am now thinking it is more likely bipolar disorder."

"The good news is that we can treat the psychosis—that is the break from reality that is common to schizophrenia, and the problem with depression—that is part of bipolar disorder, with a combination of medications. We can still get him to stable recovery, even if I still reconsider and want to make sure that we are treating the right thing. "

He was not the typical kid and his behaviors and responses to situations always were different. They said he was too sensitive but, the changes in behavior were more obvious when he was in his late teenage years. All along the psychiatrists said he had schizophrenia, and they said he had a dual diagnosis because he also had an alcohol problem. Thank God that for the last ten years he had been alcohol free. I remembered the period of severe depression when the shock treatments were done, and was glad to be over that period.

In either case, whether it was schizophrenia or bipolar disorder or both, when he was not in therapy and not taking his medications, it was like fighting a losing battle, like pouring a glass of water in the ocean and expecting to see it change. I had lived with him for so long and the cycling between a period of good mental health and poor mental health was like clockwork. This was the longest period of him not hearing voices or seeing things. The combination of the antidepressants that stabilized his mood, and the antipsychotics that kept his mind clearer of the voices and visions, was working.

Of course, I knew that people with schizophrenia have psychosis, a break from reality, and that they may hear voices other people don't hear. They also may believe other people are reading their minds, controlling their thoughts, or plotting to harm them. Sam had all of that, and I remembered it all too well from living with him and seeing patients from the emergency room, and in my experience on the locked ward during my psychiatry rotation during medical school.

I could often tell when Sam was at a tipping point. He would get a wild look in his eyes and when he spoke to you some of the things he said did not make sense. He would make connections between things that had no connection. He would become agitated, stayed up all night, and did not sleep. He did pretty well when he was on lithium and I regretted that we had to stop it because of a change in his kidney function. We had been vigilant in routinely getting the blood work for his kidney. But, at an interval when we checked, the kidney function was worse, and the lithium was stopped. That presented a setback.

On the other hand, bipolar disorder, or manic-depressive illness, usually causes shifts in mood, energy, and activity levels. Bipolar disorder symptoms can result in strained relationships with family and friends, poor job or school performance, and even lead to suicide. The persons with bipolar illness usually have periods of mania, with joy and excitement, but they also have periods of deep depression, sadness, and hopelessness. Persons with bipolar disorder may also be irritable during a mood episode. Sam had that too.

For now, I think we have Sam on the right medications. He was on an antipsychotic, and that helped with decreasing his hearing things and seeing things. He was also on an antidepressant, and that helped from him being in the dumps all the time. I decided not to worry too much if Hillpoint revisited the diagnosis every now and then to be certain that he was treating the right condition. I would rather that he does that, than blindly going down the wrong path.

"I think for right now, he is doing really well, and I plan on keeping it that way," Hillpoint said.

"Well, I have to have faith that the medications are correct. That will allow him to live as full a life as possible, but I also know the fact that he stopped drinking made a huge difference. The alcohol brought out the worse in him, whether he has schizophrenia, bipolar disorder, or both."

"I heard that," Hillpoint said.

"I only have one piece of advice for you," Hillpoint said.

"Take care of Sam. But in the meantime, you must take care of your own health too."

"Yes. Thanks. I'll do that," I said.

Felecia's dilemma

"Just be quiet, I just gave you something. Don't even try it, I just gave you something!"

I glanced up from reading the Sunday magazine section of the newspaper, and looked over the rim of my reading glasses trying to see who "should not even try it." I looked at Lyle and I looked at Felecia. I put down the coffee mug containing the Kahlua flavored coffee on the kitchen table. Lyle had just handed me the coffee that he had made from his new and fancy toy, a coffee machine. I was really digging the Kahlua flavor wafting into my nostrils and the scent was permeating the kitchen with a very pleasant smell. Was I just to be quiet, and not even try it, because they had just given me something? Huh, had I asked for something else that they did not have, or did not want to share or give me?

I was only there to read the Sunday magazine and some of the cover stories in the newspaper, chit-chat for a minute or two, and to be on my way home. I had good manners and I think that I have good sense, at least most of the time anyway. At times I might have stepped up to people wrong. But, I did not trip if they gave me the feedback so that I could change my behavior. I tried not to impose on people, and was not even trying to get into anyone's space or face if they did not want me there. No, no, I tried not to overstay a welcome, and had no intention of taking up residence in nobody's crib. Huh, so what was all this, "don't even try it" mess about?

"Just be quiet, I just gave you something. Don't even try it, I just gave you something," Felecia muttered again to herself.

Her shoulders were hunched over and she was talking into her chest. She was drinking a clear liquid from a small glass, and all of her ten fingers were tightly clutched around the glass, and her lips hovered over the opening. Was she drinking alcohol? Was that rum or vodka? I didn't even think that Felecia took a nip now and then. I never saw alcohol in their house and if they had some, they certainly never offered me any.

"Just be quiet, I just gave you something. Don't even try it, I just gave you something," Felecia said again very clearly to someone who was in the room. Only Lyle and I were sitting there. I wondered if she was talking to me.

"Oh, Felecia, I am good with the coffee. I don't need anything else," I said.

If she was drinking rum or vodka, I wondered if she had slipped some into my cup as well. I held the coffee cup with the Kahlua close to my nostrils pretending to take a sip so that I could investigate the scents, and transfer them to my brain to analyze to see if there may be something else besides Kahlua and coffee in my cup. No, the cells told me nothing else was there; nothing else had been added to the coffee in the cup. But, wasn't vodka odorless, having no smell to it? Maybe she had tossed some vodka in the coffee and I would not even know it. Would I be able to taste the vodka through the Kahlua?

I looked at Lyle who was sitting and ignoring everything around him.

"Oh, she is not talking to you," he said. "She is talking to her cough and telling it to be quiet. She just gave it something."

"Huh, huh, I had not heard her cough once since I sat here," I said.

"Oh, yeah, she is talking to her cough," Lyle jeered. "She just took, like, three different cough medicines together."

"I told her not to do that. Not to mix all those medicines together. Have you even heard her coughing? Felecia, you were not even coughing before you took all those medicines."

"Never coughed, not even once," he said.

"Gary, you are a doctor, what do you think is wrong with her?" Lyle asked.

I realized that mental illness is complex. There are many forces at work and there is not one solution to the problem. It required interventions at many levels, many touch-points. I learned, from trial and error, to ask for help, and to ask for help early. I overcame my reticence, embarrassment, and shame. I asked others what they thought. Does this even make sense to them? What is missing from the information, what else do we need to get to a logical conclusion. I wanted good information so that I could enjoy my life. I wanted you to give and to receive feedback.

Many things in life are complicated. There is rarely one simple problem, and rarely is there one simple answer. Life is a journey with many steps, and you only get to the place of recovery by taking that first step, no matter how small. However, if you are not ready, and you may never be, and even though I hope that is not what you truly want or feel, that is still okay.

I had to very calmly express to Lyle that I heard him and that I was listening.

"Lyle, you have asked me that before. Lyle and Felecia, I think the best course of action is for Felecia to go first to her primary care doctor. Felecia's doctor will get all the information and refer her to another doctor, a specialist or therapist, if she thinks that is the right place for Felecia to start. That is my suggestion."

"You can help us get the information so that we may help you. Do you want me to call your doctor for you? I will go with you, if you want," I said.

"No, no, I am not going anywhere. You don't need to come with me. I go there all the time and I have been to see all the specialists. They say that there is nothing wrong with me," Felecia said.

"That's not true, Felecia, that's not true," Lyle countered.

"The doctors made appointments with the psychiatrist and said you should go. They have done that three times already in less than one month. You always find some reason not to go. You better go to see them soon, or else," Lyle threatened.

"Gary, tell her she has to go," Lyle commanded me to tell Felecia.

I sniffed the Kahlua coffee once more and it calmed my nerves. Her behaviors were unusual. In years past, folks probably would have said she was pleasantly eccentric. She was now speaking to and commanding her cough to stop. She had some obsessive compulsive behaviors. She had some problems finishing tasks and staying on track.

When leaving messages on a voicemail machine, you could hear her reciting: "date - January 23, day—Thursday, year—2012, time—4:15 p.m.," all word for word, even before she spoke why she was calling you and who she was. She masterfully spoke a date and time stamp into any voice message that she left. I said to her, "Felecia, all voicemails will tell the person you called the time and date. The year should be fairly obvious to anyone." She did it her way anyway.

She had some very eccentric behaviors. She talked to a cough that did not exist. She told you things that you doubt were real and she made unusual connections between events that you knew were not even related. But she was not paranoid, suicidal or homicidal, and it did not appear as if she was hearing voices or seeing nonexistent things. I thought she had some learning disabilities because she could not follow simple instructions. If you gave her advice, and said it in a three step process, she would get to step one, steps two and three would never get done.

Something was not quite right with Felecia, but I could not put my finger on it quite yet. I needed to interact with her more, and she needed to go see her doctor. The primary care provider is well trained to identify and treat common mental health problems, and to refer you to a specialist, as needed. It also made for better health care if the psychiatrist and the primary care provider, pediatrician, internist, and others were in one location so that the referral process was easier. But each facility and health care organization did things differently. The path to optimal mental health had many roads, but what was important was that you get there. I wanted Felecia to get to a point where she would want to go, but that was really her choice. But, until that time, Lyle and Felecia had a dilemma begging to be solved.

Date Not, Want Not

I sat quietly at Bello Paraiso's restaurant flipping through emails on my smart phone. I should have deleted some of these messages, and saved on the telephone charges. I decided to go online to review my phone plan to verify that I was utilizing the contracted phone services appropriately.

She walked in and looked the room over. She had perfect dark brown eyes. Her skin was a flawless luxuriant chocolate. I could not guess her age but it must be somewhere close to mine. She stood there confidently surveying the room with those eyes and I waved to get her attention as I assumed she was looking for me. Here we go again on a blind date. She was Deandra's friend and Deandra thought that we might have common interests.

"Hi, I am Gary. You must be Reba."

"Yes, I am Reba, great to meet you," she answered.

"Likewise," I said.

She did not wait for me to come around to pull her chair out so that she could sit down.

"Well, I feel like I know you already as Deandra told me so much about you," Reba said.

"Yes? How's that?" I asked.

"Yes. I think she was right," Reba said answering her own question and ignoring mine.

"How so?" I repeated.

"Well, she said that you are the serious type."

"Oh, well, I guess I am," I said half-heartedly. People usually say that I am too intense, but that usually means they want to say you have issues. They don't usually say I am serious.

"...issues, that's what they usually say..."

"Sorry, I missed that?" Reba asked. "You said something about issues?"

I must have been talking out loud. I decided to "fess up" and just lay it on the table.

"Yes, people don't usually say I am serious. They usually say I have issues," I said.

"Well, I think we all have some of that. I don't know anyone alive who doesn't have some issue or another. If you are breathing, you've got to have some," Reba said with a conviction that let you know she knew what she was talking about.

Wow. I was starting to like her already. Yes, we all have issues...Then I remembered what Deandra would have said. Don't put too much out there on the first date. Don't let them see all your issues, all your stuff, all of your baggage just out there.

Airing all your dirty laundry in public with strangers was not a good idea on the first date, and probably not on the second. "So when would it be Okay?" I asked myself. Is it best if it is not too soon, or never?

I wanted to change the subject.

"Did you have any trouble finding the restaurant?" I asked.

"No, I did not."

"Good, I am glad. The restaurant is not hard to find but parking around here is ridiculous. Where did you end up parking?" I asked.

"In the lot across the street even though the fee is a little high," she replied.

"I know. I parked there too." I figured it must have been a good choice if she had parked there too.

"I usually park in a lot as I don't want to drive around looking for a parking spot," I said hoping that she would not think I was lazy.

"Yes, yes, makes sense," Reba said confirming that that was okay in her book.

"And then having to remember what time you parked to run out to put more coins in the meter," she said.

"No, I can't do that. Don't even want to do that anymore unless I definitely have to," I said.

"Yes, that's funny," Reba said. We both laughed remembering it happening once too often.

I recalled frantically dashing down to the meter to put the extra coins in just as the parking enforcer was writing me the ticket. Look at that, if only I ran faster and was not nonchalant… "Wait, wait, I got the coins, right here, please no ticket…" It was always too late as the parking enforcer, smirking, placed the ticket on my windshield. She rolled her eyes, tilted her head and seemed to say, "If you had the coins all along and knew the time was coming to an end, why did you not come and put them in before? Sometimes taking the easiest path only gets you half way there, next time, park in a lot."

We smiled as the waitress came over to take our orders.

"Hi, my name is Davita, and I will be your waitress tonight."

"Hi Davita."

"Can we start with drinks? What will you have?" Davita asked.

"Reba, how about you?" I asked.

"Oh, what's the house wine?" Reba asked.

Davita recited the name of an exotic sounding white wine from a winery I had never heard of.

"Fine, I will take that," Reba said.

"And you sir, what will you have?" Davita asked.

"You know, for now, I will take coffee and will stick to the water," I said.

"Oh, you don't drink?" Reba questioned.

"Yes, I do, but I have some work to complete once I get back home," I responded.

I was not going to explain that the reason I don't drink is that my brother drank and I was not trying to go there with alcohol at all.

Therefore, I just said, "I will drink a little wine now and then. But, I usually have to make sure I eat something first, then maybe I will have a drink."

I started to do my three-things-only on a short check-list of what I had to do for the rest of the night. I had to get to the pharmacy before it closed. I

not present

had run out of gloves at home and the bathroom cleaner with chlorine. Oh, and face masks.

Once I got back home, I had to clean up the bathroom that Sam had used, and I had to make sure I had gloves and masks. Some of Sam's medications usually made him constipated. I had given him a stool softener this morning to help him have a bowel movement. So, when I got home I was worried that the toilet seat, floor, and the bathroom rug would be soiled. So, the work was to put the mask on, glove up, and clean and clean. I would need chlorine to get the smell out, and then light the glazed strawberry scent for ten minutes, and *Voila!* The bathroom would be like new.

I hated cleaning the bathroom after those events, but pretty much I hated cleaning any bathroom, soiled or not. But thank God for chlorine and masks and scents and gloves. Yes, I was very thankful for whoever thought of disposable latex gloves.

"Dear, what will you have as your entrée?" Davita asked.

"Uh?" I responded.

I looked up at Davita. She was obviously much younger than me, and she did not look like she was from the south where that form of address is acceptable with strangers. When did that become okay to do with a stranger and a male stranger no less? Or was I just tripping?

"The waitress wants to know what you want to eat," Reba said.

I refocused for a second and then said, "Oh, how about the Giobatto? Is that the dish with the shrimp, clams, chicken, and other meats in the tomato sauce?" I asked.

"Yes," Davita replied.

"But, I don't eat clams or red meats," I said.

"So, can you take the clams and the other meats out and leave the rest of the seafood in?" I asked.

"It already comes prepared that way," Davita remarked.

"Okay, well, I guess I will take it anyway," I said.

Reba was looking at me strangely. I will just pick the clams and meats out just as I always do. I thought that Reba must be thinking, "Deandra said he was serious. He said he had issues. I told him that we all do, so that it was okay that he had issues. But, he must have some serious ones as he has drifted off once too often. I told him too quickly that it was okay that he has issues."

I smiled to bring myself back to the present company and conversation, as well as to convince myself that this date was going great.

Reba smiled back. Her teeth were a perfect pearly white. I loved the shape of her head and it was unusual in the way that her occiput jutted out in the back. Her face was oval and perfectly set with a pair of dark brown eyes that glowed mysteriously but were playful at the same time. I felt that meant she was a kind person with depth and quality to her persona. Her hair was closely cropped to the shape of her head, and she had light bronze highlights accentuating its natural black color. She worked the beautifully natural looks and dark skin that God had endowed and worked it well. Where his handiwork was a little faulty in her own estimation, she added accents, a necklace, and other highlights to optimize God's work. She smiled confidently and I secretly glanced at her again. Yes, her fashion sense was working as she implemented God's handiwork with passion and zest. God would like that.

They say that there is a divine selection out there, somewhere, for every one of us. We only need to seek and we shall find it. Maybe this was the right person that I had been waiting for. But I reminded myself not to rush headlong "where angels feared to tread." I knew that only time would tell.

CHAPTER 22

ESTHER'S UNLIKELY TIRADE

For years I've been trying to get Sam to stop smoking cigarettes. I tried to convince him to stop because of the risk of emphysema, chronic obstructive pulmonary disease (COPD), and lung cancer. In addition, he had asthma, and smoking cigarettes would make the asthma worse. On a recent occasion, his breathing was terrible, and I took him to the emergency room to get a chest X-Ray to be certain that he did not have pneumonia. Sam was short of breath, wheezing, and coughing up copious, thick, yellow phlegm. I did not have a thermometer at home, but I felt his skin, and it was moist and hot. I convinced myself that he was running a fever. He became increasingly short of breath, and I observed him excessively wheezing when he came down the staircase.

We were seen on the urgent care side of the emergency room, and fortunately, the chest X-Ray did not show anything untoward. I was concerned that the X-Ray would reveal a lung mass, not unlike the one that invaded Russell's, Esther's brother, chest. However, the X-Ray only showed over-expanded lungs. There were many areas where you saw that lung tissue was missing. Sam was starting to get a barrel chest, and I was grateful for no evidence of pneumonia. Moreover, I was glad that there were no masses, or suspicious areas, to suggest that we needed to go looking for any evidence of lung cancer.

I always hated to say, "I told you so," but smoking cigarettes damages your lungs. I knew that I had to get Sam to stop, and to get him a nicotine patch or gum to help him quit. We were still in the emergency room, and we patiently waited for all the blood work to come back from the lab. The doctor also did a nasal swab for Influenza A, "flu," to be certain that was not the culprit for the symptoms. Once all the tests came back normal, Sam was discharged home with new medications and inhalers. He was taking his medications and inhalers over the weekend, and despite that, was only slightly better. Sam still looked sick, and I was certain that he felt that way too. I would not be surprised if on Monday morning Sam refused to go to the mental health center for his appointment with the psychiatrist, and to attend group sessions.

I was still lying in bed with my eyes lightly closed, and I was ruminating about the three things on my list of activities to do today. I was on the verge of compelling myself out of bed when the screaming jolted me out of a calm mental state.

Her shrilly voice came clearly through my bedroom walls. Though my mind was at ease, my body was not. My muscles ached, and my sleep was not restful. I was still fatigued from working the night shift, and thinking about the patients that I saw during the night. I would find myself doing that often, running through the patients, their work-up, the results, and if they were admitted, or if I discharged them home. For the ones I sent home, I thought about again triple checking to convince myself that I had done the right thing. In the practice of medicine, you had to be methodical, and think things through. That learned behavior had spilled over into my personal life. My friends accused me that the behavior had taken over my social life, and that I was dull and lacked spontaneity.

"Well, we'll see," I usually responded when they asked about simply jumping up and going on some adventure.

It came again. The screaming blasted its way through the walls, and under the gap of my bedroom door, piercing the early morning silence.

"You are going today!" she screamed. She appeared to have only stopped to take a deep breath, but she screamed at the top of her lungs again.

"You're going today!" Esther said. "You are not staying in here today."

"I don't feel well, Mom," Sam quietly said. "I just don't feel well."

"Get out the bed! Get out of the bed!" Esther yelled.

Esther angrily pulled the spread off the bed. She flung it wildly behind her, and it stuttered on landing, falling limply to the cherry colored hardwood floor. The spread was really a red duvet that had striped lines running the length of it. When it was on the bed it provided cover and an ordered pattern of lines running north to south, from the head to the foot of the bed. Now that it was jumbled on the floor, the lines were zigzagging, confusing, and disorienting. The orderly design was lost, and the pattern in it was that there was no pattern.

"…but, I just don't feel well," Sam moaned.

"I don't care how you feel, I don't want to know how you feel, you are going today," she said.

Esther lunged forward to grab the pillows from under Sam's head, and she sailed them through the open door. They fluttered over the bannister and onto the first floor near the front door. She then reached in to peel away the green fitted sheet off the mattress. She underestimated her own strength as the sheet ripped at the seams and laid torn half way over the mattress. Sam still barely moved.

"…I don't feel well, I am sick…," Sam moaned. He tried to curl up more in his pajamas and tried to breathe out the words. His mouth opened slowly to speak the words out so that Esther could see that, unlike the many times before when he faked it, this time it was real and he was not feeling well.

"Get up, get up, get up! Now! If you don't get up, I will throw cold water all over this bed. Let's see if you will lie in it then. You cannot stay here today, no way, no way!"

Sam shrugged. He was not feeling well. He had lain in a cold dampness before. In fact, in the past he lay in his own urine on a soaked mattress for several hours. But that was when his mind was not clear. He felt the cold, wet, moisture beneath him then, but his mind could not interpret the liquid, and nothing compelled him to take action and to seek a dry, warm place. His mind was not foggy now. He had been taking the medications the psychiatrist had given, and he was thinking clearly. But today, his physical body was sick, he was not feeling well. Why did she not see that today? He was not physically feeling well today.

"When your ride comes, you better be ready, or else!"

Sam thought, "Or else what?" Hadn't he faced all the possible demons in his life? Clarity in his mind came and went. He had been in several psychiatric institutions. At one point it seemed as if he were trapped in a turnstile, forever going in, and never coming out. Some of the periods in the cycling were rapid, others had longer intervals. Hadn't he faced all the gargoyles? He had been bullied in school and tormented by Gasterre, his teacher. He had been cold, homeless, dirty, and hungry. Were there more trolls to vanquish? He abused alcohol and was an alcoholic. Were there other devils to fight? He had been physically assaulted, his jaw had been broken, and he also had a large healed gash, a chasm that had been so wide in the middle of his scalp from being beaten. He knew about bleeding profusely, being in pain, and being lonely, all because his mind was in the wrong place at the wrong time.

He was never good at negotiating his way out of a tough spot. He said too much, was not diplomatic, cursed, and shouted. His temper flared and the opponent's temper flared more than his. Usually, he ended up at the losing side of the war. Were there really more battles to fight? Had he not started enough of them, put himself in the middle of them, and tried to end many of them when the heat of the battle got to be too much to bear? Now, physically, one of his hands was gnarled and of little use. He needed a cane to walk and to keep balance. His knees hurt and were filled with arthritis. He was told he was likely to develop diabetes because he had too much body weight on, and he was not physically active.

Wasn't the end to all this torture somewhere in sight? He smoked too many cigarettes and now his lungs were filled with emphysema. He was sick today and not feeling well. Usually, Esther was on his side, and he could count on her being caring and protective. Today was different. Why could she not see that, today of all days, he was not feeling well? Why? Why was that?

I lay in bed, opened my eyes, and stared blankly at the ceiling. The ceiling was painted in eggshell white. The color was bright and lively. I wanted to seek refuge into the ceiling or into the mattress. I would have done anything to ignore the commotion in the next room. However, the voices got louder and the intensity of the conversation forced me to bolt out of bed. "They will figure it out," I said to myself. "Getting in the middle of a friend's disagreement was not a good idea. They are the best of friends, and I don't need to get involved."

Besides, I was going to be late for my nine o'clock appointment. I could not stop now to intervene in any drama this morning. She has coped with this for many years. I, on the other hand, only just started. She was many years ahead of me. She had a head start, first mover advantage. Let Esther figure it out. Let them both figure it.

"They are mother and son, allow them to work it out," I said to convince myself that my intervention was not needed.

Sam reluctantly went to the mental health center, and he spent three hours there going to group therapy, meeting with his licensed clinical social worker, and socializing with friends. He did not have to see the psychiatrist. By the time Sam was opening the door at home at 12:30 p.m., he looked like he had been through the wash cycle—tired and wrung out. He stumbled with his cane, and plopped down in the family room, and sat there for the next two hours.

He did not want to eat anything, even though I doubt he had eaten anything at the center. I looked over as I heard him constantly coughing.

"Are you okay? Are you wheezing? Did you use your inhaler? Is that cough dry? Are you not able to bring anything up with the coughing?"

"No, nothing comes up."

"Are you sure you are okay?"

"Yes. I am fine."

"Well, I just wanted to be sure. I have some errands to run. I will be right back."

I left him with Esther watching television. When I returned at 5 p.m., neither had moved from where they were sitting when I left.

Sam said he wanted to go to bed.

"Right now? It is only five o'clock. Well, fine. I will take you up."

At the foot of the stairs Sam handed me his cane. He held on to the railing to get up the flight. It took much longer than it normally would have, and by the time he got to landing, he was out of breath. He was breathing heavily, could move no further into his bedroom, and was slumping down in the hallway. Esther came up to see what was going on. We knew that neither one of us would be able to get him up from the floor.

"Look, we have to call the ambulance to get him to the hospital. He probably has pneumonia again. Everyone has been sick this winter."

I went back downstairs to call the ambulance, and the dispatcher told me that they would be here shortly. When the paramedics arrived, they quickly went upstairs to find out what was wrong.

"He has been short of breath and coughing all day. Here is a list of his medical problems, doctors, medications, and allergies. Please take him to the hospital. I will meet you there," I said.

One of the paramedics went back to the ambulance to get the stretcher, and they deftly got him down the stairs, and loaded into the ambulance.

The hospital was efficient, and by the time I got there, the nurse was gathering more information, getting blood work drawn, and letting me know that an X-Ray was ordered.

"It seems like you can never get enough of this place," she said.

I laughed and did not add anything else to her remark.

The test results came back quickly, and the doctor on duty told me that he was to be admitted. We had to wait for a room upstairs, and it was almost midnight by the time he arrived on the medical floor. He had more than pneumonia this time. He also had some muscle breakdown potentially related to one of the medications that he was on. Two suspected medications were stopped, but Sam still had to be in the hospital for one week. But, even after that treatment he was too weak to come home, and it made sense for him to go to rehab.

For the next three weeks Sam had physical therapy at the Bournemouth Cloisters. They did an excellent job with him so that by the time he returned home he was almost like new. He was not in perfect physical condition, but at least he could slowly climb the steps to get to his bedroom. I made a mental check, as I knew that in the not too distant future I would need to move into a ranch level home with no stairs to climb.

Some people tell me that they never plan, and that when they do plan, things always seemed to fall apart. I did not live by that philosophy. Some things could be spontaneous, and some things could not. I learned to trust intuition. If something seemed wrong, it was best to follow up intuition with information and facts. We live with uncertainty, but to reduce the chaos and stress, some things required careful planning. This was one of them. One was what to do when faced with a health condition, and another was how to prepare for future life changes that you knew would certainly come.

Sooner or later, neither Sam nor I would be physically able to climb the steps at home. I wasn't crossing the bridge before I got to it. But, I had to plan for it, and to figure out how to get across once there.

Dressed to Impress

Felecia looked at herself in the mirror, glowed with pride, and beamed back at the reflection in the mirror. She loved the way the dress glittered with its shininess. She suppressed a giggle as she started to feel giddy from the brilliance of the beads and the way the dress perked up her face, neck, and body. She needed the jolt of uplifting that the dress gave her because recently her spirits were low.

"Wow!" she exclaimed silently to herself.

The patterns of the silver leaves on the platinum colored dress reminded her of how leaves clung to pure white snow just after the first snowfall. If you concentrated and focused long enough on the leaves you could even see the tiny dew drops formed on the leaves as they lay in their snowy winter wonderland. The water dew was like tears frozen in time, invisible except to the most discerning of eyes. Felecia knew a thing or two about tears. She had cried too many yet, no one seemed to notice. Maybe, it was better that way, hidden and camouflaged by the surrounding beauty of the snow, leaves, and trees.

"Yes, this was perfect," Felecia thought. The dress constantly sparkled.

"Ooh, ooh, I simply love this dress," she squealed with delight.

Felecia ignored the fact that the skirt was a bit too tight.

"Oh, oh, ooh, I think this will do. Yes!" Felecia purred. She spun on her heels and ran down the stairs to show the dress to me.

This was the second week that I had stopped by to pick up the Sunday newspaper from Lyle. I was heading to sit down in the kitchen when Felecia appeared at the foot of the staircase. You could see the stairs from the kitchen as this set of stairs landed near the hallway between the kitchen and the family room.

Lyle, Felecia's brother, was true to his usual form. He rolled his eyes upwards. He began to huff and puff, and you could see the steam forming in his nose. His face became a sarcastic snarl, and I held my breath in anticipation of the venom that he was intending to spew out. I did not want to be in his way when the poisoned words started to sputter out. Like unanticipated projectile vomiting, there was certain to be flecks of vomit on items and people that were simply anywhere near the location. You would be unnecessarily soiled, the innocent bystander in the casualty of an unnecessary war.

Lyle was so impatient with everything, and I wondered about all the constriction to the blood vessels to his heart and brain as he was huffing and puffing. Was all that venom really necessary? Please don't give yourself a heart attack or stroke over this, I thought. I just don't think it is worth it.

The snarl was still there. But, he tried to distract himself and to ignore Felecia by playing with his new phone.

He had just bought an Icicle or Popsicle or Ice-cream or whatever. This was his new phone. Lyle was smart and tech savvy. He bought all the new gadgets as soon as they became available. He was the go-to-guy for all technology questions. Invariably, he would be one of the persons you'd see standing in line at 4 a.m. to buy the latest equipment.

"Look, it has 4G. Yeah, this is great. Look, it has this "app" and that "app." And the response time is remarkable," he chortled. Lyle kept blurting out the new "apps" and going on and on about all the applications that were on the new phone.

He barely lifted his head to look up when Felecia came down the steps.

"Hey, Gary, do you like my dress?" Felecia asked.

"Yeah, it looks all right," I said.

"Is it new? Is it something new that you bought?" I asked.

I surveyed the kitchen counter for a second time. I had already looked as soon as I had walked into the kitchen. I did not see a wooden counter block of knives there.

"Uh, did I miss it the first time? Are you sure there is none there?" I asked myself.

The kitchen was the most brightly lit room in the house. The wall was sunflower yellow, and at first I thought that the color was too bright for a kitchen. But, I grew accustomed to its effect on livening up the house and lifting my spirit. It was like waking up to a tropical morning with lots of sun and light. It jolted the senses and forced me to smile. I thought about painting my kitchen that color to prevent seasonal affective disorder.

The countertops in the kitchen were laminate. They were not granite, marble or Corian. I found that to be unusual for a house of this size and caliber.

"Uhm, if I lived in this house I would think about replacing those laminate counter tops. It was too retro and it was like living in the past and way back to the sixties." I thought. I wanted to live in the present and look towards a happy future. I wanted consistency and I craved harmony. I did not want to be in a kitchen with walls that shouted out to me to feel alive, and then look down at countertops that wanted to pull me back to the past. I wanted to see a matching yellow countertop or at least one that was complementary. That would keep the feeling of sun and light and aliveness as you started the day and sat down to drink your first cup of coffee. It would be a super perfect way to start each and every day.

Good. They must also do the same thing. No matter where I've live with Sam, I always made sure that there were no knives around. I did not think he would be aggressive and use it on anyone. He had not done that before. Except for the time that I left the knife out that night, only to come down stairs to find Sam saying that he wanted to kill himself, I had not made that mistake twice. Prevention is better than cure, and better be safe than sorry, I reasoned. Why take unnecessary chances? It was not worth the risk.

I always recoil whenever I see a knife block perched on a countertop. My reaction was based on a muscle memory that created an involuntary flinch and reaction because of what Sam had done that morning. I had also seen too many violent movies, and watched too many breaking news stories to feel comfortable with knives around.

I knew that Sam tried to slash his wrist before. For some reason his medications were not working and I suspected that something had changed. Maybe he was not taking the medications, or he had reached a plateau and was slowly sliding off a slippery slope. However, at the same time, he was diagnosed with pneumonia, and was eventually hospitalized for it. He was saying that he could not take it anymore, and that he was not going to make it this year. It could have been his not taking the psych medications, combined with the medical illness and the pneumonia. He was restless, irritable, and obviously not well. I could not tell what the specific problem was at that point in time. But, once he brandished the knife, I asked him to put the knife down on the counter, and told him to calm down.

I took him to the emergency room and the workup showed that he had pneumonia. He was in the hospital for about a week being treated with intravenous antibiotics. I had gone home and removed all the sharp knives from the house. From that point onward, I did not keep sharp knives visible, and I never kept a block of knives propped upon the kitchen counter. I would not do that now, and I knew that I would never do that again even if I lived alone.

I glanced around the kitchen a second time. I wanted to be certain that I did not miss any knives, or a knife block the first time in my surveillance.

"Good, no knives," I said, breathing a sigh of relief.

"No, it's my mother's," Felecia said triumphantly.

On that pronouncement, Lyle jerked his head up and away from playing with his new phone.

"What? What?" he asked.

Now he was definitely interested in what Felecia was saying. Before that he had completely ignored her and me. The new play thing dangled in his hand.

"Oh, yes, it's Mommie's dress," Felecia cooed.

"Mommie just told me to wear it," she added.

"I just saw her and she told me to put it on and wear it out," Felecia said confidently.

"How could she do that Felecia?" Lyle asked.

"How could she do that?" he asked again with the phone still dangling.

"Mommie is dead," he dryly stated. There was no hint of emotion in his voice.

"Well, I just saw her and she told me to wear it," Felecia boldly said.

"Well, I don't care what she told you, go take it off," Lyle commanded.

"Why? I am wearing it to the party," Felecia said.

"No, you cannot," Lyle said.

"Why?" Felecia defiantly asked.

"Gary, tell her why she can't," Lyle said, now backing away from the conflict.

"Felecia, is that your mother's dress?" I asked.

"Yes," Felecia replied.

"Well, why are you wearing it? Why are you wearing it now?" I asked.

"Well, I need to clean out her closets anyway," Felecia answered. "And, I need a dress," she added.

"Besides, my mother never liked to see anything good go to waste," Felecia said, adding more reasons to vindicate her actions and support her argument.

"Oh, God," I said quietly under my breath.

"Felecia, your mother has been dead for two years," I said.

"Why would you wear her dress? Don't you have one of your own that you could wear to the party and that would fit the occasion?" I asked.

Felecia shrugged and ignored the question. She wanted to talk about what she wanted to talk about. In her mind her behavior was logical. She was not willing to be questioned and challenged to see if her reasoning and logic would remain intact. Felecia wanted to wear that dress and that was that. Nothing was going to dissuade her.

"Well, I need to clean the closets out," Felecia said.

"And I just saw Mommie and she told me to wear it," Felecia bravely said.

"Yes, but if you are cleaning her closets out, why do you need to wear that dress?" Lyle asked. He was gaining enough confidence to ask the question directly. He would not run away from conflict this time. He asked the questions and, I supposed, was ready to hear an answer that he did not want to hear.

"Why not give the dresses and clothing away?" I asked.

"Why not take them to a women's shelter or somewhere? Anywhere," I added.

Felecia shrugged and did not answer directly. She was not going to make any commitment to take the clothing anywhere. Felecia said that she saw her mother, and that her mother told her to wear the dress. Lyle challenged her asking how that was possible when their mother was dead for more than two years now. I vaguely remember the service. I was not afraid of death or dying. I considered it a part of life, just as I thought birth was a part of life. But now I hated to look into caskets at a funeral. I had not looked into the casket at the service to confirm that their mother was in it. After working in the emergency room for so long, I did not want to see another person's body after they had died. I did not want to look and I did not want to see a lifeless body. But, I was certain that their mother passed away and was buried. I was not the only one there. There were many people there. I had not imagined it. It had to be at least two years.

I decided that I could no longer completely ignore that Felecia might be having visual and auditory hallucinations. The last time I was here, Felecia was talking to her cough, and commanding her cough to stop. I knew that there were enough signs already that something was not quite right. Felecia had periods of derailment, delusions, disordered thought and disordered content, visual and auditory hallucinations, paranoia, and some sense of persecution. My intuition said that Felecia and Lyle were not ready to have that conversation. But, she really needed to go to her doctor.

My sense was that pushing blindly headlong along this line of discussion might not be a good idea right now. I reasoned that I had to figure out what was the best strategy to approach this topic in a way that was meaningful and helpful to her. I was a doctor by profession, but first I was their friend. I quickly needed to figure out a way to talk about what I was observing. I did not want to bring up a subject and risk that I would alienate them. And who knows, was I opening Pandora's Box? The timing had to be right, but it also had to be immediate. With the limited information that I had, my assessment was that Felecia was not a physical threat to herself or to anyone else. There was no clear and present danger. But what if I was wrong? I needed to find a way to encourage Felecia to voluntarily talk to her primary care doctor, or to go directly to a therapist and psychiatrist. Time would be of the essence, and I needed to figure that out sooner than later.

I don't think that it was only that Felecia was grieving the loss of a parent and was just stressed out. I was not an expert on grief, but two years seemed like a long time to still have those emotions so raw. Maybe wanting to wear her mother's dress was a way to hold her mother's memory close, and to feel her mother's presence.

"Felecia, why not donate the dress and the clothes?" I asked again trying to get to the root of what was going on with her.

"Well, I like the smell of it," Felecia said.

"Her scent is still in it, and I can remember how beautiful she looked in this dress. It makes me happy to be in it, and I think of all the good times we had together. I feel her presence still lingering in it, you know?" Felecia said.

No. I really did not know. But, instead I said, "Yes, that's probably a good thing. But wearing it might not be such a good idea."

"I mean, for you to wear her dress to the party," I said, trying to correct myself, and to clarify what I was trying to say.

"See, see. I told her she needs to see a shrink," Lyle interjected.

"No, I don't need to see a shrink. You need to see a shrink," Felecia countered.

"Gosh, Lyle, just hold on for a moment, will you?" I interjected, trying not to let him escalate a conflict before we had a chance to talk and to figure it out.

"Well, Felecia, talking to a therapist has helped many people share what's on their minds. It's good to talk to your doctor about your physical health, as well as your mental health."

"Whatever. But, I know you do not need to be wearing Mommie's dress to the party. After all, everyone will see you in it," Lyle said.

"That's not right," I said.

"Yeah, listen to Gary," Lyle said. He was thinking my saying "that's not right" was meant for Felecia.

"Yeah, he is used to crazies. That's why he can deal with you, Felecia. Listen to Gary," Lyle said.

I looked across the room at him. Lyle was always so indelicate. He usually evaded conflict, but when he decided to approach the subject, the words may be minced, indirect, if not incorrect.

"I am used to dealing with crazies?" I asked myself. "Is that what my life had become, dealing with crazies?"

"Yeah, you know. She's got what your brother's got," Lyle said.

"Schiz-koid. Skits-whatever, you know, Gary, you know," he added to clarify his thought.

"What? How's that?" I asked.

"I thought your mother said Felecia had "water" on the brain after she had an ear infection as a child? Was that not the case?" I asked. "Anyway, that's what you told me."

"Felecia probably had bacterial meningitis as a complication from an ear infection," I said.

"Yeah, she had that too."

"Water on the brain," Lyle snorted.

"Schits-koid-whatever. That's what she's got," Lyle emphatically repeated.

"No," I said, directing my comments to Lyle.

"My brother has schizophrenia," I said.

"Yeah, so isn't that what I just said?" Lyle asked.

"And there should be no stigma about it," I said.

"Just like people have diabetes, high blood pressure, and asthma, and take medication for it without people turning up their noses, they should be able to talk about their mental health problems, take their medications, and not feel like they are being judged, tried, and convicted over something they are born with," I said.

"Well, we need to get Felecia tested for that," Lyle said.

"She ain't right, I tell you. She ain't right," Lyle said repeatedly as if we had not clearly heard him the first time he said it. He apparently wanted to make certain that somebody in the universe was listening and heard him. There is good communication, and there is bad communication. And that is better than no communication at all. This time his communication needed some tweaking, and we needed to find a way to help Felecia, and help him at the same time. But at least this was a start to get them both at the table to get a conversation going. *did they need help?*

I suspected that he was correct, that a mental health concern was an issue, even if his proclamation did not come out in a manner that was politically correct. I knew that getting Felecia to go talk to a health care provider was not going to be easy. I breathed deeply again trying to focus my mind and my body into a more calming equilibrium.

Did I not just see a block of knives on the kitchen counter when I walked in?

Or was I over-concerned with a non-issue?

Marta's tears

Even a house with a sturdy foundation will develop cracks in it. I watched the house appraiser looking at the jagged cracks in the foundation. The largest one was near a window, and he forcefully knocked on the window sill and the crack several times with the red and gold handled screwdriver that he held in his hand. He knocked on the serpentine break to see if it would move or break way. I worriedly looked at him and he saw the concern in my eyes.

"Oh, that is nothing to be alarmed at now. We will see how deep the fault in the concrete goes when we go inside. This house has a solid concrete foundation, and all houses here do, but they still develop cracks in the foundation. Once I get inside the basement, I can then tell you if there is something you should be worrying about. If the core is solid, this house can withstand any tempest, any storm, any wind, or any disaster."

"The trick is to be certain that the visible fault line is only on the surface. It rarely goes to the core of the house to destabilize the foundation. If you build a strong foundation to the core, you should be all set," he said.

Therefore, with that advice, I thought about when Esther's brother, Russell, died. She had relied on him to take her to visit Sam at the psychiatric hospital. Russell was a heavy cigarette smoker. By the time he decided to go to the doctor because he had constant coughing, had lost a massive amount of weight, and had shortness of breath simply walking across the room, the mass had invaded half his right chest. The doctors completed all the testing and lung biopsy and confirmed advanced lung cancer. In less than one month he was dead.

At Russell's funeral, I silently sat and blankly stared at Marta as she was crying uncontrollably. Marta was one of several cousins. She was at the brink of bawling her poor eyes out of the sockets. Marta was seated in the middle pew on the right side of the church, and she chose to take the first seat of that row. As relatives and guests walked up and down the aisle, they were forced to brush past her, and there was no choice but to see her sobbing. She strategically placed herself in the perfect seat, so that you saw her as you went up and back down the aisle from the receiving line.

Marta cried, stifled a sob, sighed, heaved, and sniffled, as her body shook with emotion. It was hard to ignore it as the pew itself was shaking by her rocking back and forth. How any of us could keep our composure seeing her like that was a mystery to me. I imagined that soon her tear ducts would run dry, and I hoped that nothing else would come out from them. I held my breath and prayed for the point when she would have no more tears left.

That did not happen soon enough, and Marta kept on bawling. It wasn't that I did not want her to express her feelings; it was only that I had no clue that she had them.

Something actually moved her. Even as a child, Marta always gave you that "tough as nails" and "stronger than living steel" persona. She was very sarcastic, and she got to her point quickly, usually in two seconds flat. She was razor sharp, and in every interaction with her you walked away feeling the cut. You would be left bleeding, but, what was nice about her is that she always warned you that you were about to be cut. You never saw the prick or slash, but you felt it. In her presence we all expected a frontal assault as she did not stab you in the back. If you chose to be around her at all, she would tell it to you as plainly as she saw it. There were no niceties, and it all came out straight with no chaser.

Don't put on your rose colored glasses in Marta's presence. She grabbed them off your face and stomped on them. She shot directly from the hip, and if you started a discussion, and she had any inkling that you were sugar coating anything, she would strip the sugar off so that you would lay there with everything out, raw and bare. Nothing ever seemed to faze her, and she took negative comments in just as deftly as she dished them out. We all knew that she had weathered the many storms of life. But, you would never know it, and I am sure she would never tell it. She was calm, cool, biting, sniping, and she was pure concrete and steel. We called her Ice-lady when she was not around to hear it. But, that was only a façade, because today, you saw that she had a heart. She really had emotions, and somewhere behind all the wall of steel a tender heart was hidden. She was not impermeable and she had at least a button or two. It was unbelievable to finally see that something could get to her, and break her down just as it would to the rest of us.

I looked up to see some of Russell's children now standing at the podium on the altar. Some said that he loved them and was glad to be in his life. Others skirted the subject, and only said that they remembered him doing this, or not doing that, and if only they had more time. Whether any of that love was reciprocal was not frankly stated. None of them touched or hugged each other. I wanted them to hold hands while standing there, but they did not.

Victoria, one of the daughters, read a searing elegy—a poem lamenting the dead—that she had written for him. Everyone in the church was stunned into silence from the grief that we shared. Most of us suppressed our crying, as we felt the emotions, but we tried to keep them locked away inside. Like Marta's crying, the overwhelming grief was a slippery slope, so that if we showed any emotion at all, it would take us to a place where we were not prepared to go. Esther was one of the few relatives who had a dry eye in the place. She said that she had her complete breakdown before the funeral, and was now prepared to turn the page, and to move on. She always said, "Give me my roses when I am alive so that I can cherish them, for when I am gone, I won't know that you even cared."

What do you say at moments like this? There were no words, no thoughts, no emotions, no cards, no letters, no flowers, and no acts of kindness that could ever fully describe the deep pain of losing a sibling, or any loved one. You thought you knew, but unless you have walked in those shoes, how could you really know how it felt? Could you understand a pain that you have not endured, not walked, and not lived in?

Pastor Dolane stood up to bring the church service to an end. He was tall and thin and his hair was balding in the middle. There was a deep dimple in his left cheek, and a thin scar like a river's tributary running into it to pool with others and flow back outwards. He was always cheerful. He wore a red robe embroidered with gold trimmings along the lapels, and he stood up confidently and bellowed over the crowd.

"This person, Russell, was a gift given to you," he said.

"It was a blessing and not a curse. It is how you choose to live with what is given to you that will make it your blessing."

I glanced at Marta, she had stopped crying. I looked at Esther, and her eyes were closed. She seemed lost somewhere in that interspace between grief and acceptance. I also felt calmer by the fact that they both appeared at peace now, and it helped to calm my own emotions.

"…most of us always say, Lord, why me, Lord, why me? And the Lord answered, my child, why not you?"

Marta opened her eyes and a single tear clung to her cheek. I quietly hoped that she would let the tears and emotions freely flow if she needed them to. It was good to know that showing that you had feelings was not a sign of weakness. We all experience some sort of pain and emotional distress in our lives, and it really was how we used that pain, that struggle, that curse, to get to a better place, and make that experience a blessing.

Pastor Dolane and the choir stood up, and he led them in singing the "The Lighthouse."

> There's a lighthouse on a hillside
> that overlooks life's sea.
> When I'm tossed He sends out a light,
> light that I might see.
> And the light that shines in darkness now
> Will safely lead me on
> If it wasn't for the lighthouse
> This ship would sail no more.
>
> Oh, if it wasn't for the lighthouse
> Then where would this ship be?

———

The appraiser was there because I was thinking of selling my house to go to a ranch with one level. Therefore, he came to give me an estimate of what to expect. After he completed his assessment, he slowly got up. He was kneeling to examine the basement floor, and he wobbled for a moment when he stood back up. However, he steadied himself before answering the questions that I had asked.

"Was the house's foundation in trouble? Did the crack in the concrete go beyond the surface? Was the house at risk because of it, would it topple over at the earliest sign of trouble?"

"Oh, my knees," he said.

"I have been doing this too long, and I am starting to get arthritis in my knees," he complained.

"You will be fine," I said to reassure him.

"That break in the foundation is nothing as it is only the surface. It doesn't go to the core of the foundation. You are on solid ground, solid concrete, solid as a rock."

I remembered Marta that day as she opened her eyes, and more tears began to fall. She too was solid as a rock. What I also observed that day was only a small crack in the façade, and it did not even go anywhere near the solid core foundation.

CHAPTER 23

A SHORE IN SIGHT

I t had been a while since Sam and I had gone anywhere on vacation. In fact for the last several years, Sam had been in and out of the hospital so often that we never seemed to find the time. Some friends suggested that we go to Martha's Vineyard on a day trip that was organized by Northwood Tours. The bus was leaving from the commuter lot at six o'clock in the morning, and I bought the tickets deciding to do something fun for a change.

We arrived without incident at the lot on time, and I was amazed that everyone was so chirpy so early in the morning. The other passengers all look like they were retirees, and they were happy and laughing and appeared as if they had no cares in the world. The driver left the commuter parking lot and took Interstate 95 North towards Providence, Rhode Island. He then followed the highway routing to Cape Cod crossing over the Bourne Bridge to get into Woods Hole, Massachusetts.

The driver let us off at the Woods Hole terminal, and we boarded the ferry to take the short ride over to Martha's Vineyard. We had taken a wheelchair for Sam because I knew that he could not do much walking. I was glad that Liam, Bette, Esther, and Ermelinda were with us because no single person could manage pushing Sam on the ferry and on the streets all day. Besides, as we took turns, each of us would be able to take in the sightseeing at different stages.

Upon boarding the ferry, the uniformed attendant told us that we should have informed them ahead of time that we were traveling with someone needing assistance. If we had, he would have allowed us to get on the ferry with the wheelchair ahead of the more able-bodied passengers. It was a pleasantly warm July summer day, and the sun was beating down on us energizing our bodies. The attendant was the epitome of a sailor. He was physically fit and he obviously spent more than his share of time in the sun. He was well tanned, and his white shirt and khaki pants were crisp and light, and was intended to keep him cooler in the hot sun.

The ferry had passengers of all ages going to the island, and everyone was dressed in summer clothing, capris, brightly colored blouses, shorts, and T-shirts. They all seemed to be looking forward to spending the day on Martha's Vineyard for the day, or for a couple of weeks. I plopped down in the nearest seat close to the exit sign. Sam said he wanted something to drink, so I got sodas for all of us. I was glad that they served beverages, sandwiches, and snacks on the ferry.

The ferry takes only forty-five minutes to cover the seven miles from Woods Hole to Martha's Vineyard. Once I was comfortably seated, the quiet rocking of the ferry started to lull me to sleep, and I closed my eyes and dreamed about relaxing on the island for the day. We would have had no time to go to the beach, as this would simply be a ride on a tour bus to get a whiff of what the island had to offer. It was an enticement, and I promised myself that was a good entrée, and I would come back next year to explore the places of interest.

We disembarked the ferry at Oak Bluffs, and boarded an old school bus. I could not get the wheelchair down the aisle, so I placed it from the back emergency exit door. The bus driver was a musician who did this work part-time.

He was an excellent ambassador for the island, and in fact, he was an ambassador for life itself. He laughed loudly, and told us so many jokes that just listening to him was worth the trip. He knew everything about the island, and named every morsel of it. He gave us the history of the gingerbread houses on Ocean Avenue, and the original uses of the bed-and-breakfast places that now lined the streets.

If he was this jovial driving a bus, I anticipated what it was like listening to him playing his instrument, the saxophone. He said he drove the bus, not only to keep his mind and body active, but to explore the unfamiliar. He loved working on the tour bus and meeting different people. It was not that he did not have that experience on his many travels. But, this was like taking his message to a different audience, in a different format, and in doing so he found unexpected inspiration. He said that everybody had a story to tell, and he was happy to share his.

At the end of two and one half hours sightseeing from Oak Bluffs to Edgartown, he let us off at the Information Center and bus stop at Church Street. We pushed Sam down Winter Street to a nearby deli, and I took the lunch orders and went inside while Sam, Liam, and Bette sat outside under the shade of a tree and looked at passersby. A lot of people rode by on bicycles towing a lunch basket or a child propped on a high seat. I wanted a vegetarian sandwich and everyone else opted for chicken salad sandwiches. I gave Sam his sandwich and his soda. I was very happy to see him having a conversation with everyone. His speech was clear and coherent. He was obviously happy, and so was I. We needed a change of scenery, and the day and weather was perfect for that.

I was glad that Sam decided to come with us because most of the time he refused. I was glad that this blend of medications was working to help him be engaged with life. To be as whole as possible: leisure activities, fun with family and friends, and a vacation day. If you do not try to enjoy your life you become like stagnant water. Water was essential to life, but when it was stagnant, it became foul and destructive. It wore away stone, rotted wood, and even when it stood still the plant life that grew in it would not appreciate it after a while. If there were no new water, the minerals exhausted, the nutrients absorbed, and it became hard and useless. Eventually, the plants too resented it as they withered away and died. Stagnant water was never any good. Water's life was to keep moving, to nourish, to create, and to carve out a new path and design. Water wanted to be fluid, nonresistant, flexible.

I loved looking out at the water, the rivers, the seas, and the oceans. It washed away my stress, and cleansed me so that none of it could stick to any part of my mind and body.

I was more than happy to see that Sam was smiling, and I was ecstatic even if it had taken a lot of work. He was stable on his medications, and it was for at least six months now. When you live with someone with a mental health condition, you truly begin to appreciate life. Everything. All the small things that life has to offer, every day is a good day. I made it a good day because tomorrow was not promised, and I didn't know what tomorrow would bring.

A Prayer for Sanity

Aida did not enter the pool and she paced along the edge as I swam the length of it. She was saying, "kick, kick, kick." Aida was my swimming instructor, and she was extremely patient and encouraging.

"What are you afraid of? Kick, kick, kick…," she encouraged.

"You can do it. You know that you won't sink, and that you can breathe," she added.

"Stop holding your breath like that, slowly let the air out in the water, and when you need to, turn your head and breathe. Breathe and kick. Kick, kick, kick…You can do it and you won't sink to the bottom. We have already worked on floating so you know that you won't sink. You can do it."

I knew that I could swim. I had been swimming against the tide for a great part of my life, and I felt that I swam upstream and downstream, in shallow water and in deep. Many times, I held my breath, afraid to breathe, but I always kicked to stay alive.

When I stopped my medical career to come back home to take care of Sam, I just simply wanted to get him off the streets. I knew that as soon as he was discharged from the hospital, he would be homeless again. I knew that was a burden that he could not bear, and one that I could no longer watch in silence. I simply could not do it any longer as we were both suffering emotionally.

The decision was not an easy one, and when I started I did not know what I had volunteered to do. But, in the more than ten years that he has lived with me, I think that I have learned more about myself and others. I drew on the life skills that I learned from working in the emergency room, and I realized that half of the persons coming to the emergency room have a mental health concern that needs attention. If I had not gone through this experience with him, I would not have learned to breathe, to choose a path, to follow your heart and instincts, freeing your mind and enjoying your life. I learned that we should not wallow in self-pity, but to look up, and to look out, and to be the best that we can be.

"Breathe, Breathe, Breathe…"

I kicked to keep moving in the water and I breathed to stay alive. You too should swim upstream or downstream and you should breathe to stay alive.

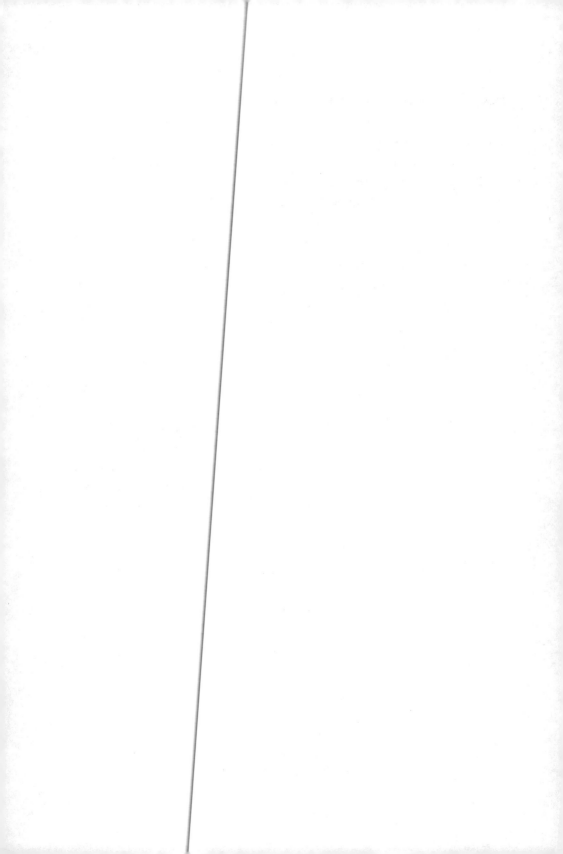

EPILOGUE

I was looking forward to my last twelve-hour shift before I would have a long weekend off. As I sat in the fishbowl where the doctors sat to do their charting, I heard the emergency medical system radio go off. Most likely it was another Code Blue. Neissa, the charge nurse today, picked up the phone, and listened to what the ambulance crew was bringing in. They wanted to have Med Control, and wanted to have a doctor stand by to hear what they were doing, and to ask permission to give some medications.

Neissa looked directly at me through the glass of the fishbowl, and she waved me over.

"Med Control is now here, please go ahead," Neissa said.

"It's Med Control, doctor number 123," she added. All the doctors were assigned a number to document in the EMS system when they provided the medical control advice for treatment. We did not use our first or last names, and using a number system was easier than spelling out our names.

The Code Blue was a young man that was not breathing and was found by his family. The ambulance crew had arrived ten minutes after his family had last seen him. He was found on his bedroom floor and he was unconscious. They placed him on the heart monitor and put a tube into his mouth to control his breathing. They checked for a pulse and it was slow and erratic. There were no obvious signs of trauma to his head or body, and the crew said they could not get a blood pressure reading. The crew said they lost the pulse, but it looked like his heart still had some kind of electrical activity on the monitor. The young man was somewhere near the brink between here and there.

I sniffed for the smell of lilac. It was not there.

The ambulance crew started the resuscitation, and was fervently working to bring him back to life. Maybe this was a drug overdose, and I knew the crew would speak to the family. They would scan the room and see what was around him, as maybe there was a bottle of pills or alcohol lying there next to him. The resuscitation would continue on the way to the emergency room.

"What's your estimated time of arrival?" I asked.

"We will be there in ten minutes," the crew said.

I hoped that this was a Code Blue that we saved, as there were too many traumas, too many Code Blues, and too many lives lost.

"Okay. Continue what you are doing, but call back if there are any problems before you get here. We will see you in ten," I said.

I knew that this was the emergency room, and we had to do what was fundamental. First and foremost is safety, to protect our patients and ourselves. Every person that came through those doors had a family or a friend, someone who cared and wanted to know that they would be all right. Someone cared and someone should. This was fundamental.

I saw too many Code Blues and saw many people come through the emergency room doors. In one way or another, some of them have an underlying mental illness. This affected what they thought about the health care system, and it affected how they interacted with their health care providers, their families, friends, and community.

I prayed for a day when we removed the taboo around the discussion of mental illness, and removed the stigma of a mental health diagnosis. I looked forward to a time when we had a fundamentally rational and comprehensive approach to mental health problems, and I dreamed for that to include emotional support for the family.

I prayed for safety and to have fewer traumas, fewer Code Blues, and fewer lives lost.

I only wanted to be free. When I volunteered to do this work to live with my brother, I had no clue what I was doing. But, in the process, I learned a lot about him, a lot about all of us, and a lot about everyday people trying to get to a place for their optimal mental health. Once I anchored myself with love, I learned about compassion, tolerance, and our common humanity. I learned that life is filled with rainy days and unexpected storms, but that there is always the calm and sunny skies after each and every storm.

Anchor yourself in love and you can survive it all.

Free your mind and enjoy your life!

TIP BOX 6

1. Take a day vacation and enjoy yourself
2. Anchor yourself in love, and with loving people all around you
3. Always go to the root of your stress and write out the actions that you will make to calm your mind. Keep it on your desk, or a visible space to remind yourself what you will do to get there

DBT

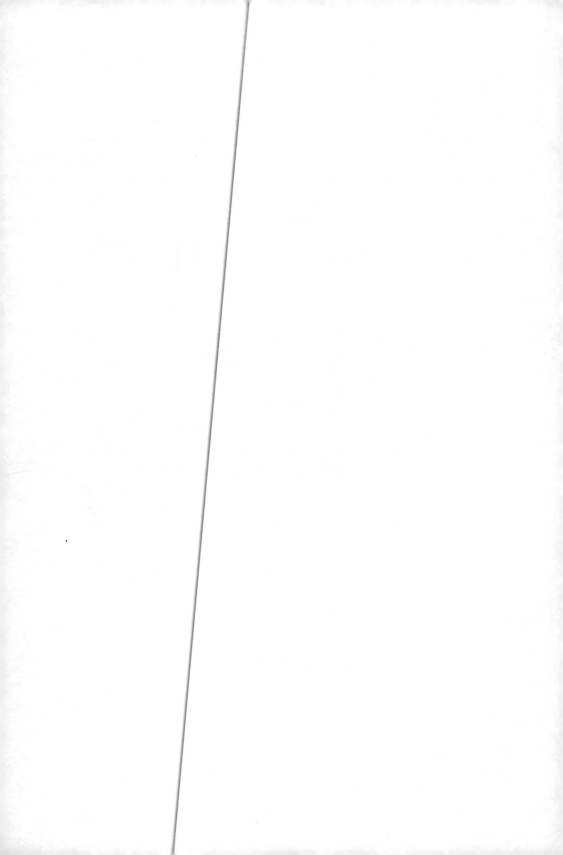

ABOUT THE AUTHOR

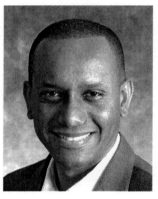

Gary Rhule is a board certified Internal Medicine physician and healthcare management consultant. He worked for many years as an emergency room doctor where many persons are affected by physical illness, as well as mental illness. He is interested in improving the mental health system, removing the stigma of mental illness, and closing gaps in health disparity. He was born in Jamaica and has lived in the U.S. since his teenage years. He now lives in Connecticut with his family.

To learn more about the author, please visit **www.garyrhule.com**

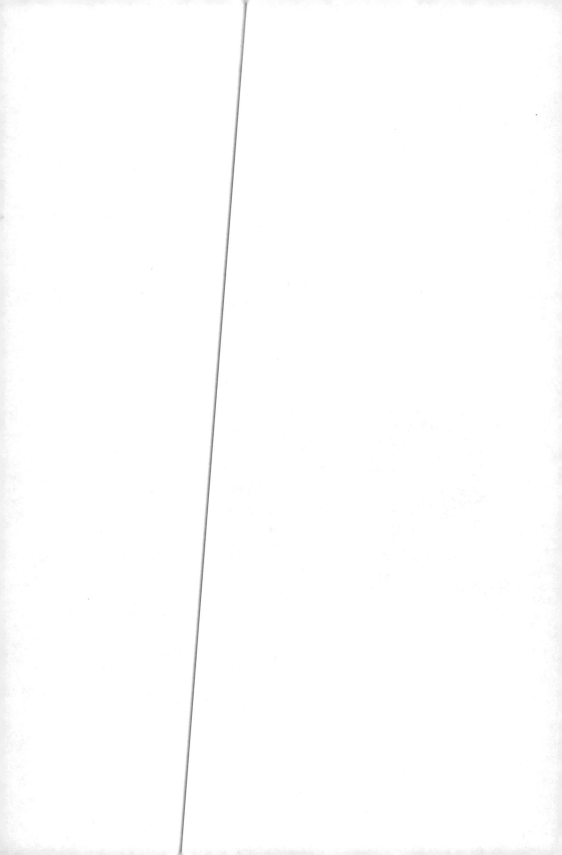

Conservatorship p.138, 140, 141
Anxiety disorders are most prevalent p.199

CPSIA information can be obtained at www.ICGtesting.com
Printed in the USA
BVOW03s1654190614

356832BV00003B/109/P